D1357401

CURIOSA
A miscellany of clinical and pathological experiences

FRONTISPIECE

The theme of some of the histories in the three books of this series might be 'How not to . . .'—How not to be a doctor, How not to be a specialist, How not to be a patient, How not to be an administrator, How not to be a pathologist, How not to . . . Of course, it is of only a very small part of our corporate experience that this is the theme: but however small, the part is important enough casuistically to bear consideration. The photograph chosen for the frontispiece may be thought to symbolize a certain negativist attitude; some interpreters may recognize in it a vulgar pictographic paronomasia—if they do, they are in error, for that is not its purpose. In fact, the picture is here only to illustrate one inapposite way of involving the laboratories in our common approach to complete diagnosis.

What we see here is a radical mastectomy specimen as it was on arrival at the laboratory, stuffed in a jar several times too small, so that the volume of fixative solution that remains is so insufficient that it could not have adequately preserved more than the relatively trivial proportion of the tissue that it had effective access to. The result was that the interior of the breast was far gone in autolysis, and the microscopical detail of the tumour such as should not justify attempted diagnosis.

These wide-mouthed jars of tough glass, with easily fitted and leak-proof plastic screw caps, are still the ideal container for surgical specimens, provided the jar is large enough to contain ten times or so as much fixative solution as the specimen displaces.* The more modern disposable plastic or waxed card pots may be cheaper, but their usual opacity is a disadvantage, sometimes even facilitating the loss of small pieces of tissue—parts of endometrial curettings, or of needle biopsy specimens, for example—by the pathologist who for

---

* While formalin and other preservative fluids are likely to remain with us for quite a few generations, the hospital that is lucky enough to be allowed the means to have a well organized and reliably staffed delivery service can best translate its surgical specimens from theatre to histology laboratory in their fresh state. This means *fresh*, not delayed half an hour, not exposed to contamination, not left standing in a hothouse atmosphere in the

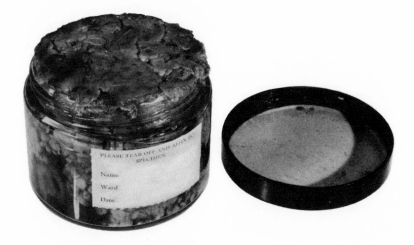

the moment has given in to the pressure of a day's experiences or, rarely, who is just casual in his work. Clear plastics, which should be an answer, seem often to be too brittle for jars of these materials to withstand the strain of conveyance within hospitals.

Whoever may be responsible for supplying specimen jars to operating theatres, clinics and wards has to appreciate that a reasonable margin (say, fifty per cent) ought to be allowed for use above the intended purpose. The glass jars with their sound and firm fitting lid are just what is needed for the consultants' sugar, the SHO's jam and the night super's Earl Grey . . .

By the way, the specimen jar takes many other forms and may contain specimens other than those intended. This is a topic to be illustrated in another volume in this series (*Memorata,* Chapter 43) . . .

---

operating suite. The advantages of being able to permit the pathologist or his well-trained aide to dissect and preserve the specimens under conditions that are best suited to accurate diagnosis, photography, demonstration and—occasionally—permanent preservation are too often the unattainable goal: yet they are advantages that from time to time can save a life or spare a patient mutilation. Accurate diagnosis needs dissection free from confusion or sequestration of significant observations by distortion through shrinkage and hardening in unnatural orientations, the almost constant accompaniment of the usual careless habit of simply immersing the excised portion in fixative without preliminary (skilled) opening, cleaning and protection from shrivel and twist.

An occasionally invaluable bonus of the ideally presented fresh specimen is the better chance of being able to obtain useful microbiological investigation when, even unexpectedly, this turns out to be particularly relevant to the diagnosis or treatment of the patient's condition.

Curiosa

A MISCELLANY OF CLINICAL AND PATHOLOGICAL EXPERIENCES

collected by

William St Clair Symmers *Senior*
Pathologist, Charing Cross Hospital
Professor of Histopathology in the University of London
at Charing Cross Hospital Medical School

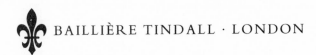 BAILLIÈRE TINDALL · LONDON

Baillière Tindall
7 & 8 Henrietta Street, London WC2E 8QE

Cassell & Collier Macmillan Publishers Limited, London
35 Red Lion Square, London WC1R 4SG
Sydney, Auckland, Toronto, Johannesburg

The Macmillan Publishing Co. Inc.
New York

First published 1974

ISBN 0 7020 0470 7

*Published in the United States of America by
the Williams and Wilkins Company, Baltimore*

*Printed by William Clowes & Sons Limited
London, Beccles and Colchester*

Introduction

This is a collection of unusual clinical and pathological experiences, presented for the interest of doctors engaged in any field of Medicine (and, with no base motive, occasionally for their entertainment). It is an anthology, mostly of case histories: only the essential observations are included, in the hope of making each account concise and readable, though neither inaccurate nor lacking any important detail. Each 'chapter' records simply the facts that combined to make its topic noteworthy: comment is included only if comment seemed desirable, or if the temptation to comment was irresistible.

References to 'the literature' are deliberately few. This is not a reference book—only an occasional publication, interestingly relevant to the theme, is noted. A few of the cases have been reported elsewhere: this is noted in the text, the references being given at the end of the chapters.

Scientific merit may not be claimed for a compilation like this and is not its aim. Equally, the book is not intended to be light-hearted. Yet Medicine has its share of light-hearted moments, and to disguise this would have been artificial. I hope that nothing in these pages will offend any reader.

Most of the chapters concern patients whom I have met since becoming a medical student in the Queen's University of Belfast, almost forty years ago. Whoever reads these accounts will realize that I owe very much to colleagues who allowed me to share their experiences: their skill and humanity, often inseparable, have greatly outweighed mistakes and human failings, and it is not churlish to record some of the latter among a small representation of the former. I owe no less to the patients, too, and to their relations, for théy have so often helped understandingly and with interest when it seemed necessary to explore their histories, sometimes painfully: such delving into things past must at times have seemed irrelevant, even impertinent, yet it was exceptional for the information to be kept back.

No case has been included against the wishes of the patient or of the patient's family, or of any doctor. Several colleagues asked that their names should not be mentioned: this seemed at first likely to make it impossible to refer to their patients' cases, but eventually most of the histories have been included, largely thanks to arguments in favour of publication put forward by some of these doctors themselves. Enough of them would stay anonymous to make it best, though regrettable, to name none at all of those colleagues whose help has made this compilation possible. I can express my thanks only in general terms to them all, humbly and with warmest appreciation of what I owe.

The story in most cases is told in the manner of its development. The reader who will accept a challenge to do better in interpreting the history or the findings ought, if he can, to ignore the illustrations before they are referred to in the text.

A few chapters relate clinical or laboratory errors. These are recorded in no primarily critical sense—we all make mistakes in practice, whether we work directly with patients or deal with specimens in a laboratory. Our mistakes are often harmful to our patients and may be mortally so: we are fortunate that this is not oftener the case, and it is indeed remarkable how often our patients, like ourselves, are none the worse for our shortcomings. Putting some of these on record, some of mine among them, may have a prophylactic value and should not in itself be thought disgraceful: hiding what we have done wrong is seldom justifiable.

Some of the cases are examples of what are classed, often with some contempt, as 'small-print diseases', the sorts of clinical rarities that are seen seldom, once or never in a professional lifetime. But some doctor has to be the first to recognize the individual patient's rare disease: and to the patient the print is large enough and its significance worrying. This book is not a compendium of 'rare' conditions: yet I feel no apology to be needed for including some, some even that are unique, among these *Curiosa*—no one who lives by the microscope neglects the reality of the physically small and its importance in the larger scheme of things. So, I hope that the lacing with 'small print' will be acceptable, even if such cases are unlikely to be repeated in the reader's own practice— his 'small print' will be another story . . .

*   *   *

The content of this volume and of the two that may follow it has been discussed, and often constructively criticized, by medical audiences in many countries, when *Curiosa et Exotica* has been a lighter topic among the more substantial subjects of lecture tours. Indeed, it is some of those who were my hosts on such occasions who have suggested that these histories might be collected usefully into a book: this explains why, eventually, and rather to my surprise, I sit at five o'clock of a winter morning in England in 1973 typing this introduction to the finished volumes. I have enjoyed putting these books together: I hope that they may be both enjoyable and interesting to others.

Miss P. M. Turnbull, head of the Department of Medical Illustration, Charing Cross Hospital and Medical School, prepared the Frontispiece and Figs 30.8, 30.9, 30.12 and 32.1 for *Curiosa*. Except for Figs 19.1, 19.2 and 36.1, all the other photographs in this book are by Mr R. S. Barnett, of that Department. Mr Barnett's work on the illustrations to the published version* of a selection of *Curiosa et Exotica* presented as my Presidential Address to the Section of Pathology of the Royal Society of Medicine, London, in 1969, gained him the Lancet Trophy for medical photography in 1971.

My friends Mr F. D. Humberstone, Mr K. R. James and Mr J. K. Turnbull helped invaluably with the technical preparation of most of the specimens illustrated. 'And so the job got done, nowise else . . .'

Northwood, Middlesex   W. St C. Symmers
November 1973

Publisher's Disclaimer

The author has altered or omitted the names, physical descriptions and whereabouts of all patients whose cases are described in this book, in order to ensure their privacy. Similar steps have been taken to prevent possible identification of the medical and professional staff concerned. In addition, prior approval to report these cases has been obtained.

---

* *British Medical Journal,* 1970 (December 26), *4,* 763–7.

Contents

PHOTOMICROGRAPHY

Unless stated otherwise, all the histological preparations illustrated were paraffin sections of tissue fixed in formol saline (ten per cent formaldehyde). Most were cut at about eight microns. Standard technical procedures were used in every case, the material examined being without exception acquired in the ordinary course of the practice in diagnostic histopathology of general hospital laboratories.

The photomicrographs were made with a Carl Zeiss 'Ultraphot II' equipped exclusively with Zeiss optics. This apparatus, invaluable in providing photomicrographic records of the highest quality both in the course of research and for teaching (in the widest sense of the word), was bought for the Department of Histopathology of Charing Cross Hospital and Medical School by the Board of Governors of the Hospital in 1966 and has been kept optically up to date by the generosity of the Council of the School and of certain benefactors whose wish is to be unnamed. It is a pleasure to thank the Board, the Council and the good friends of the Department for this practical support.

1 Actinosimulation: Actinobacillosis[1]

A medical registrar, who—through overwork—had neglected the early symptoms of his illness, was admitted to his own ward with lobar pneumonia. After at first improving rapidly on treatment with penicillin, the condition failed to clear completely. Two months after the start of the illness he still had opacity of part of the middle lobe of the right lung, and now there was evidence of abscess formation.

The affected lobe was removed. Histological examination showed chronic suppuration and considerable fibrosis. In the haematoxylin–eosin sections there were several conspicuous structures in the pus that the pathologist interpreted as colonial 'grains' of actinomyces (Fig. 1.1). The trainee pathologist attached to the department was working for a postgraduate diploma: his chief suggested that the specimen offered a good opportunity to practise histological methods of staining the actinomyces. The trainee began with a Gram stain: not finding the expected Gram-positive filaments, he assumed that he had over-decolorized the sections. Further attempts, appropriately controlled, confirmed that there was no Gram-positive material in the colonies, which in fact consisted of tightly clustered masses of small, Gram-negative coccobacilli (Fig. 1.2). The histological diagnosis of actinomycosis was changed to a presumptive diagnosis of actinobacillosis.

The patient developed a postoperative pneumonia of the left lung. Cultures of his sputum gave a heavy growth of an actinobacillus, apparently identical in its cultural characteristics, biochemistry and antigenicity with *Actinobacillus actinomycetem-comitans*. No actinomycetes were isolated, despite many attempts; and no filaments of actinomyces were found in the sputum. Interestingly, the actinobacillus grew rather better in the presence of therapeutically attainable concentrations of penicillin than on the same medium without it. The organism was sensitive to chloramphenicol: the pneumonia, which was thought to have resulted from a spill-over of infected exudate during the lobectomy, cleared rapidly when this drug was given.

Comment

There was no evidence that the registrar had ever had actinomycosis. It seems likely that his initial illness was a straightforward lobar pneumonia, and that actinobacillosis developed as a secondary infection.

The actinobacilli rarely cause disease in man. This is true even if certain organisms that are not now generally regarded as actinobacilli are still included among them. For instance, the glanders bacillus, *Loefflerella mallei,* which seldom infects man, was sometimes known as *Actinobacillus mallei*. And *Streptobacillus moniliformis,** the cause of a form of infective erythema and polyarthritis (Haverhill fever), typically acquired through taking contaminated food (particularly milk), is sometimes referred to as *Actinobacillus muris* (the infection may also result from a rat bite†).

The 'True' Actinobacilli. Actinobacillus lignieresii causes 'woody tongue' in cattle, an infection liable to be confused with actinomycosis ('lumpy jaw'), but lacking the latter's tendency

---

* It was in cultures of *Streptobacillus moniliformis* that L-forms of bacteria were first discovered (see page 126).

† Streptobacillary rat-bite fever may not be distinguishable clinically from the rat-bite fever that is caused by *Spirillum minus*.

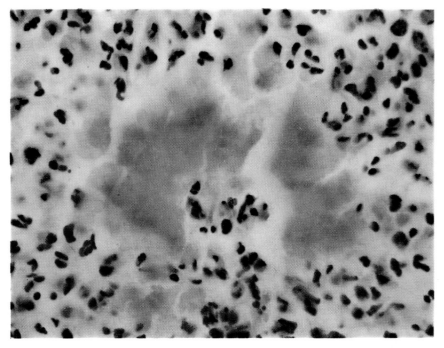

Fig. 1.1. The structureless-looking body, part eosinophile, part haematoxyphile, that occupies most of the field has the appearance of a colony of actinomyces, complete with peripheral zone of 'clubs'. The surrounding cells are part of the suppurative reaction. See Fig. 1.2 also.

Haematoxylin–eosin × 630 *From an 'Agfachrome' transparency (same size)*

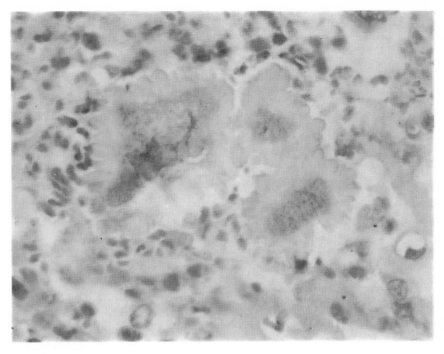

Fig. 1.2. The Gram preparation shows no Gram-positive material in the colony, the central part taking only the red counterstain because it is an aggregate of the Gram-negative coccobacilli that caused the infection, *Actinobacillus actinomycetem-comitans*. If this had been a colony of actinomyces, the fine, branching, Gram-positive filaments characteristic of that organism would have been readily seen (as they are in Fig. 1.4). The yellow appearance of the peripheral 'clubs' is due to their affinity for the iodine used in the Gram procedure.

Gram stain   × 630   *From an 'Agfachrome' transparency (same size)* to invade bone, and spreading in the lymph stream rather than in the blood. Human infection by this species is of doubtful occurrence.

Actinobacillus actinomycetem-comitans, as its name indicates, has usually been found in association with actinomyces (*Actinomyces israelii*) in lesions of actinomycosis in man. Its pathogenic significance in such cases is debatable. Its relative insensitivity to penicillin, which (in 1974) is still widely used in Britain in treating infection by *Actinomyces israelii*, may be one reason why the cure of actinomycosis with this drug requires such large doses over so long a period. The occasional association of penicillin-resistant bacilli with actinomyces has

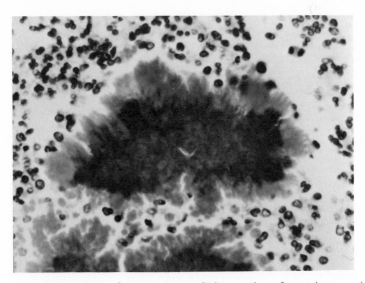

Fig. 1.3.   This colony of *Actinomyces israelii* in a section of an actinomycotic abscess may be compared with the colony of the actinobacillus in the coloured illustration (Fig. 1.1). The central darker part of the colony in both instances consists of the micro-organisms, the paler peripheral zone of clubs mainly consisting of protein and other matter precipitated at the surface of the colony. In a haematoxylin–eosin preparation the filamentous structure of the actinomyces cannot often be made out (compare with Fig. 1.4).

Haematoxylin–eosin   × 450

been an argument for treating actinomycosis with tetra-cycline, to which actinobacilli are generally sensitive.

In infected tissues, the true actinobacilli are known occasionally to form colonial granules, or 'grains', very similar to those of actinomyces. The clinical importance of distinguishing actinobacillosis from actinomycosis has been mentioned already—penicillin, so likely to be used to treat the latter, has little or no action on the actinobacilli. Confusion of the grains of actinobacillosis with those of actinomycosis can be avoided if care is always taken to look for the fine filamentous structure that characterizes the colony of acti-nomyces—Gram staining is still the simplest and most reliable means of demonstrating it (Figs 1.3 and 1.4).

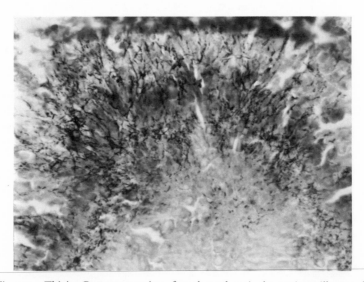

Fig. 1.4.   This is a Gram preparation of another colony in the specimen illustrated in Fig. 1.3. The filaments of the actinomyces are seen well. In this colony, as often is the case, the organism has not given a positive Gram reaction in the central region, presumably because there is no viable growth left in that older part. The vesicle-like structures in the core of the colony are in fact cross sections of the iodophile 'clubs' (compare with Fig. 1.2).

Gram stain   × 450

However, grain formation is a comparatively rare feature of actinobacillosis. Most cases of pure actinobacillus infection do not show this feature. Infective endocarditis is by far the commonest manifestation of such infections.[1] Interestingly, there is a haemophilus, *Haemophilus aphrophilus*, that is very closely related to *Actinobacillus actinomycetem-comitans* and causes similar infections, but without any so far recognized tendency to form grains in the tissues, and only exceptionally associated with actinomycosis.[1] The importance of distinguishing this haemophilus from the actinobacillus is that it is much likelier to be sensitive to penicillin than the latter; both organisms are usually sensitive to chloramphenicol, tetracycline and streptomycin.

References

(1)   Symmers, W. St C. (1967) Curiosa et exotica—a selection of clinicopathological observations of unusual presentations and manifestations of familiar diseases (Case 2). *Journal of Postgraduate Medicine, 13* (October), 143–50 (The Dr Dhayagude Memorial Lecture in Pathology, 1967, delivered at Seth G. S. Medical College, Bombay, on 7 March 1967).

(2)   Page, M. I. & King, Elizabeth O. (1966) Infection due to *Actinobacillus actinomycetemcomitans* and *Haemophilus aphrophilus*. *New England Journal of Medicine, 275* (July 28), 181–8.

2 Actinosimulation: Staff Staph[2]

A surgical registrar, who—through overwork—had neglected the early symptoms of his illness, was admitted to his own ward with acute appendicitis. Appendicectomy was performed, without drainage. Histological examination showed gangrenous appendicitis with no unusual features. During the week after the operation he had some evening fever and remarked on pain in the lower part of the abdomen. On the seventh day a tender lump was felt in the right iliac fossa: at laparotomy, the omentum was found to have sealed off an abscess beside the caecum, adjoining the stump of the appendix, which had not been infolded. The abscess was evacuated. The surgeon recovered.

Sections of a piece of the abscess wall taken during the second operation showed what seemed to be typical colonies of *Actinomyces israelii* (Fig. 2.1). However, no filamentous organism was found in Gram-stained films of pus from the abscess. Instead, when the 'sulphur grains' that were present were crushed and stained they were found to consist wholly of clustered Gram-positive cocci. Actinomycetes could not be cultured and aerobic cultures gave heavy pure growths of penicillin-resistant *Staphylococcus aureus* of the phage type that was an endemic trouble-maker in the hospital. Re-examination of the histological specimen showed that the haematoxyphile core of the actinomyces-like granules had a non-filamentous structure: in Gram preparations it was clearly seen to consist of masses of Gram-positive cocci.

6

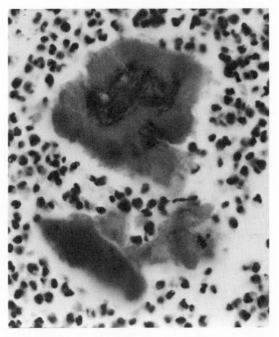

Fig. 2.1.   If this picture is compared with Fig. 1.3 (page 3) it will be clear that there is no significant difference between the appearances. Yet this is a colony of *Staphylococcus aureus*, as was shown by Gram preparations and cultures.

Haematoxylin–eosin   ×450

Comment

The actinomyces-like bodies were colonies of staphylococci—the condition was that known as staphylococcal botryomycosis or staphylococcal actinophytosis, which are elegant-sounding names that lack pertinence. This condition may be associated with a high titre of agglutinating anti-staphylococcal antibodies in the patient's serum. It seems possible that the staphylococci are agglutinated by these antibodies in the inflammatory exudate, but survive and continue to multiply.

The often radially patterned eosinophile zone round the colony can be shown to consist partly of fibrin, partly of globulin and partly of polysaccharides. Immunofluorescent staining with fluorescein-labelled anti-staphylococcal antiserum confirms the presence of staphylococcal antigens both in the core of the colonies and in the peripheral zone.

The eosinophile material covering the colonies is comparable to that round colonies of actinomyces, round single fungal cells in some cases of sporotrichosis and other fungal

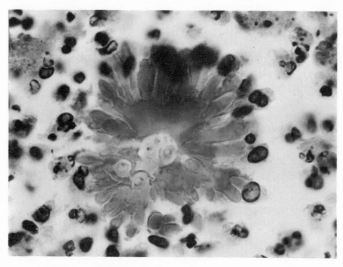

Fig. 2.2.   This is a candida 'asteroid'. so called because the hyaline eosinophile material that has formed round the fungal elements has a more or less distinct radial orientation, producing a star-like pattern. The nature of the eosinophile material is debatable: sometimes it includes fibrin and gammaglobulin, clearly derived from the host's resources, and polysaccharides that are probably the product of the fungus—the perhaps too facile interpretation is that it represents an antibody-antigen reaction between fungus and patient. Similar asteroids are seen in sporotrichosis, coccidioidomycosis and some other fungal infections;[2] they may form round metazoan ova in the tissues and sometimes even in relation to inanimate foreign bodies of various sorts.

The asteroid illustrated is from a case of septicaemic infection by *Candida albicans* in a heroin addict. Several fungal cells are seen (the rounded structures within the hyaline mass).

Haematoxylin–eosin   × 700

infections (accounting for the appearance of the 'asteroids' in these conditions; Fig. 2.2), and sometimes round ova or dead metazoan parasites.

While staphylococci are the usual cause of 'botryomycosis' or 'actinophytosis', other bacteria may be responsible:[3] the actinobacillus was mentioned in the last chapter (page 2)—others include pseudomonas, proteus and streptococcus.

References

(1) Symmers, W. St C. (1967) Curiosa et exotica—a selection of clinicopathological observations of unusual presentations and manifestations of familiar diseases (Case 4). *Journal of Postgraduate Medicine, 13* (October), 143–50.
(2) Symmers, W. St C. (1972) Histopathology of phycomycoses. *Annales de la Société Belge de Médecine Tropicale, 52*, 365–88.
(3) Greenblatt, N., Heredia, R., Rubenstein, L. & Alpert, S. (1964) Bacterial pseudomycosis ('botryomycosis'). *American Journal of Clinical Pathology, 41* (February), 188–93.

3 Actinosimulation: Bubula (Pliny)[1]

A lawyer, middle aged and otherwise very fit, had been inconvenienced for some years by a recurrent peptic ulcer on the lesser curvature of his stomach. He was by nature a heavy eater, enjoying his food when his ulcer was not too troublesome. Paradoxically, it seldom bothered him when he was working under pressure, particularly in court. When eventually it perforated, it did so without warning, when he was gathering his papers in the courtroom immediately after the successful end of a long and exceptionally demanding case.

The perforation was closed by a purse-string suture, and as much exudate as possible was aspirated from the abdominal

cavity. Five weeks later, in spite of the prophylactic administration of penicillin throughout that time (it was 1948), a
second operation became necessary for drainage of a large
residual abscess in the lesser sac. Part of the abscess wall was
sent to the laboratory for culture and sectioning.

The cultures, aerobic and anaerobic, were sterile. In
contrast, the haematoxylin–eosin sections showed several
clumps of irregular, fragmented, eosinophile material in the
purulent exudate (Fig. 3.1). At first these were taken for
colonies of actinomyces: their unusual appearance and uniform eosinophile staining were interpreted as due to the
organism being dead, killed by the antibiotic, with consequent loss of the haematoxyphile filamentous structure
characteristic of the usual actinomycetic granule. However,

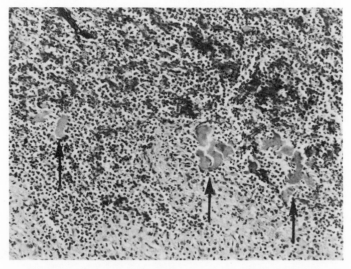

Fig. 3.1. Part of the wall of the abscess, with organizing granulation tissue
below and pus in the cavity above. The three arrows indicate eosinophile masses
that are rather less eye-catching than in the original section (what a pity colour
illustrations are so expensive). The darker material in the purulent exudate is
fibrin. See Fig. 3.2 also.

Haematoxylin–eosin   × 120

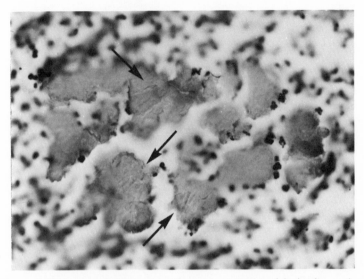

Fig. 3.2.   The arrows indicate areas where cross striation of the hyaline eosino-phile material may be seen. As is so often the case, the two-dimensional limitation of the photomicrograph deprives us of the advantage that the fine focussing adjustment of the microscope provides in enabling features to be more clearly seen that in a single plane cannot be well shown. Despite that, this picture shows the key diagnostic appearances reasonably well. Once the possibility that these structures were pieces of meat was appreciated, it was a question of time before this could be proved: the proof came in the form of specific immunofluorescent staining, using a fluorescein-labelled anti-beefsteak antiserum to make the point (perhaps a procedure in the event only justified by the experience it gave in methodology).

Haematoxylin–eosin   × 420

careful focussing with the fine adjustment of the microscope showed cross-striation (Fig. 3.2): it was realized that the structures were fragments of meat—perhaps pieces of the barbecued beefsteak that was the main course of the patient's lunch a couple of hours before his ulcer perforated, five weeks earlier.

Comment

Oddly enough, as one may confirm sometimes in the contents of an appendix abscess or similar lesion, cooked meat—

perhaps especially meat that has been charred—may remain long recognizable, in spite of exposure to leucocytic and other enzymes.

Reference

(1)   Symmers, W. St C. (1967) Curiosa et exotica—a selection of clinicopathological observations of unusual presentations and manifestations of familiar diseases (Case 3). *Journal of Postgraduate Medicine, 13* (October), 143–50.

4 Actinosimulation: Fibrin

A nurse had been troubled since childhood by occasional discharge from one ear, a result of chronic otitis media following scarlet fever. Her parents belonged to a religious group that did not believe in medical attention: because of this she did not have expert treatment until she became old enough to make her own decisions.

At 21 she became a student nurse. Soon afterwards she had an exacerbation of the middle ear disease. When this had subsided she was advised to have a mastoidectomy: she declined because it would have interrupted her training. For several years she had no trouble other than slight deafness on the affected side and occasional otorrhoea. Then, when she was just past her thirtieth birthday, a severe head cold was followed by persistent discharge from the ear, earache and increasing deafness.

Treatment with antibiotics had less than the expected effect on these symptoms. Troublesome headache, dizziness and some disorientation led to neurological examination, which suggested the presence of a lesion of the temporal lobe of the brain on the side of the otitis. Suspecting an otogenous brain abscess, a surgeon opened the skull and in the temporal lobe found a mass from which he aspirated thick, opaque, yellowish fluid and some small fragments of tissue. No organisms were found in stained films or on culture of this material. Histological examination showed the fragments to consist of inflamed and necrotic brain substance: haematoxyphile branching filaments found in and round inflamed blood vessels were taken to be hyphae of *Actinomyces israelii* (Fig. 4.1).

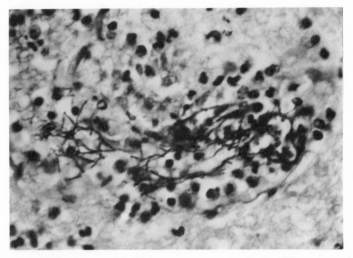

Fig. 4.1   The haematoxyphile filaments are seen quite clearly. What may not be quite so evident is that they are within the confines of a blood vessel in the inflamed and partly necrotic brain tissue. These are fibrinous filaments, not the mycelium of actinomyces as was originally thought. In retrospect, it is hard to accept that there might be some justification for mistaking these filaments for anything other than the fibrin threads that they were to prove to be. Isn't it the retrospective realization of the obvious that sometimes is so useful a mentor?

Haematoxylin–eosin   ×550   *Black-and-white reproduction of an unrepeatable colour transparency* (the only histological preparation that showed the appearances so clearly was rashly put out at a demonstration to a learned society: one of the members was not so learned in her use of the microscope, and racked the oil immersion objective through the slide).

Outcome. Three days after the operation the patient died in coma. The PM showed extensive fresh haemorrhage into the lesion, which proved to be a necrotic glioblastoma. There was no infection of the brain or meninges, and no evidence of any intracranial complication of the middle ear disease, which was a straightforward chronic suppurative otitis media of long standing.

Re-examination of the biopsy sections showed that the filaments were fibrinous: there was no evidence of actinomycosis or any other infection.

If . . . If the original histological diagnosis of actinomycosis had been checked at the time by examining Gram-stained sections, it is likely that the pathologist would have recognized that the filaments were not as strongly stained as filaments of actinomyces should have been.

If this observation had been made, the sections might have been examined more thoroughly. Then the single small focus of atypical cellular proliferation that was eventually found would have been seen before her death and the possibility of tumour considered. But this would have made no difference to the outcome.

Comment

Fibrin tends to precipitate in filamentous form in the blood after death (or in biopsy specimens) unless enzyme action is stopped promptly by putting the specimen in fixative solution. Sometimes, as in this case, the fibrin filaments, when produced through the action of cerebral thromboplastins, are more haematoxyphile than fibrin usually is. Their haematoxyphilia in this case was too marked to be typical of actinomyces, and this ought to have raised a doubt about the interpretation.

5 The 64 000 Dollar Vermiform[1]

A schoolboy, aged 10, was admitted to hospital with a day's history of nausea and mid-abdominal pain. He had vomited once, was constipated and had a temperature of 38° centigrade. He looked ill. There was rigidity of the abdominal muscles, particularly in the right lower quadrant, and there was marked tenderness at McBurney's point. His tongue was dry and white. No Koplik's spots were seen (there was an epidemic of measles at the time) and he had no rash. Acute appendicitis was diagnosed.

The parents refused to allow an operation, and asked that the boy be treated with antibiotics and sedation, a regimen they had read about in one of the monthly digest magazines. Their doctor talked them into having a second opinion. Another surgeon and a children's specialist then saw the boy: they agreed with the diagnosis and the need for immediate appendicectomy. Fifteen hours more went by before the parents agreed to the operation, after still further consultations. They warned the surgeon that the operation would be undertaken against their judgement and that accordingly they would hold him responsible for anything that might go wrong. Their solicitor drew up a contract to this effect—the surgeon refused to sign it and, after a cutting exchange with the child's parents, went ahead with the operation.

The abdomen was opened through a paramedian incision. The appendix, which was gangrenous, was enclosed by the greater omentum. Appendicectomy was performed without drainage. The appendix was put in formalin and sent to the laboratory for examination, the usual practice of the hospital. The pathologist's report, worded by his trainee assistant but signed by himself, read:

> Gangrenous appendicitis following obstruction by an impacted faecolith, with Warthin–Finkeldey giant cells [Fig. 5.1], pathognomonic of measles, in the lymphoid tissue. No other noteworthy features.
>
> *Summary*: MEASLES IN GANGRENOUS BUT OTHERWISE NORMAL APPENDIX.

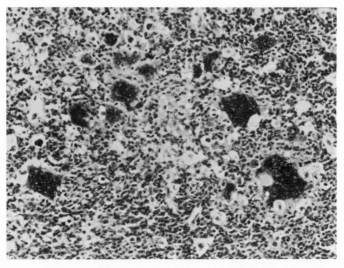

Fig. 5.1.   Looking carefully at the dark structures, they can be seen to be multi-nucleate cells with so many nuclei that nuclear substance makes up virtually the whole of their matter. These are the pathognomonic Warthin–Finkeldey cells of measles, seen here in the lymphoid tissue of the child's appendix.

Haematoxylin–eosin   × 140

The child's progress was very satisfactory for a week after the operation, in spite of the development of the typical measles rash on the second day. On the eighth day, a faecal fistula opened in the laparotomy wound, and within the next few days three small abscesses formed in the tracks of the skin sutures and gave rise to persistent sinuses. A week later, a subcutaneous abscess appeared some centimetres from the laparotomy wound and had to be incised: this led to a further sinus, and others soon formed elsewhere in the affected quadrant of the abdominal wall.

One day, seven weeks after the appendicectomy, the staff nurse, changing the dressings, saw what she thought might be 'sulphur granules'—colonies of actinomyces—in the discharge from one of the sinuses. Until then, examination of the exudate, which had included anaerobic as well as aerobic cultures, had not suggested actinomycosis. Further granules were found and quickly identified as actinomyces—*Actinomyces israelii* was cultured from them.

Review. The diagnosis of actinomycosis established, the histological sections of the appendix were re-examined. No colonies of actinomyces were found, either in the original sections or in sections cut from further blocks prepared from the preserved specimen. No filaments were seen in the haematoxylin–eosin sections from any of the blocks; but in Gram-stained sections, short isolated lengths and small tangles of filaments were seen in a few blocks, including two of the three originally sectioned (Fig. 5.2).

Progress. The boy was treated with large doses of penicillin over several months and recovered completely. When the diagnosis of actinomycosis was made there was clinical and X-ray evidence suggesting an incipient intrahepatic abscess: this came to nothing, the signs disappearing early in the course of treatment with penicillin.

Claim. He was in hospital for nine months altogether. Shortly after his discharge home his parents, on his behalf, claimed damages against the hospital's management, the surgeons, the

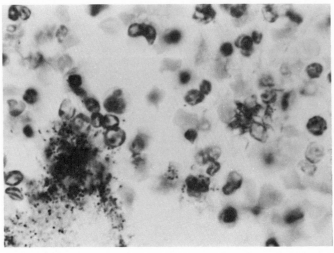

Fig. 5.2.   To the left, below, is a large cluster of bacteria, both Gram-positive cocci and Gram-negative coliforms: in the context of this case they may be neglected. What is important, what was initially overlooked, though there to be seen (if only Gram preparations had been made) (and, being made, had been conscientiously examined), is the little tangle of actinomycetous filaments at the centre of the right half of the field. Actinomycetous? Yes, that can probably be a justified interpretation, even in the absence of hindsight (see text); but are they a pathogenic actinomycete? And, if they are, are they pathogenic in this case? With hindsight, yes—without it, perhaps yes, perhaps no . . .

Gram stain   × 1100

paediatricians and the histopathologist. The sum was well into the five-figure bracket, in British money. They based the claim on the failure to diagnose actinomycosis immediately after the appendicectomy and attributed to this failure the length of his stay in hospital and his consequent loss of the advantages throughout that period of being at home and at school.

Counsel's opinion was sought on the practicability of contesting the claim. He advised negotiating an out-of-court settlement, in view of the undeniable circumstance that the eventual Gram staining had shown the means to the correct diagnosis to have been available at all times from the moment of the appendicectomy, and that therefore the pathologist had been negligent in not obtaining and examining Gram preparations before making his original report on the appendix.

Learned counsel further criticized the pathologist for closing the original histological report with a summary that was ambiguous, contradictory and injudicious, and that could be held to be maliciously frivolous and incompetent.

Outcome. There were many unpleasant discussions between the management of the hospital and the doctors concerned and their advisers. The management, represented by an unfortunately chosen trio of its members—an anti-doctor politician, an anti-clinical doctor and an anti-university businessman—fought openly and behind the scenes (and understandably, by their standards) to have the whole liability put on the doctors concerned, particularly the pathologist, as he was employed by another authority and had only an honorary contract with the hospital.

In the end, it was agreed that the boy's parents should be offered a quarter of the sum that they had claimed, still a very large amount. The solicitor's letter to this effect, addressed to the parents' advisers, was awaiting the final consideration of the chairman of the hospital before being posted, when, totally unexpected, a letter came from the claimants stating that they had decided not to proceed further in the matter, subject only to the payment of their legal costs.

This was an anti-climax. The final bill was a small fraction of what it might have been. Before it was settled, however, coercive steps were needed to silence the litigious clamour of those in some authority who wanted to press the hospital's luck, contest payment of costs and counterclaim for the management's expenses.

The abandonment of the litigation had its cause in an event happier than most in this history. Three months after leaving hospital the boy sat an examination for entrance to the school that his parents had set their heart on his going to: he passed, leading among the candidates and gaining a valuable scholarship. Acknowledging the worth of the facilities that the hospital had arranged so that their son could continue his education while a patient, they dropped their claim.

Sequel

The pathologist, having learnt a lesson in pathology, felt that the affair had ended reasonably well. He was soon to discover that it wasn't quite over for him.

The hospital management board, which had a few medical members (most of them not practising), ordered a post mortem on the case. The outcome was that the pathologist, who had not been invited to the enquiry, received a directive that henceforth all appendicectomy specimens in cases of acute appendicitis were to be serially sectioned throughout their length and that alternate sections were to be stained with haematoxylin–eosin and by Gram's method so that in future no case of actinomycotic appendicitis would be overlooked.

After a predictable first reaction to this bidding, which was the recommendation of a medical scientist on the board who had often denied medical omniscience, the pathologist did some sums with the chief technician in the histopathological laboratory. After confirming the results of these calculations by consulting with cronies in other institutions, he wrote to the management, their obedient servant, accepting their directive. His acceptance was expressly conditional on the management providing him with the means to implement their requirements:* the space to accommodate an additional histopathologist to examine the sections, two additional senior histological technicians and two juniors to prepare the sections, and the funds to buy the additional microscopes,

---

* Figures from the pathologist's memorandum in support of his conditions are set out at the end of this chapter (Appendix 1).

microtomes and other equipment for the additional staff to use . . .

Sequel of the Sequel. The management studied the document, deliberated, thanked the pathologist for his cooperation and asked him to regard his obligation to implement the directive as 'indefinitely in abeyance for the time being'. In fact, he was left to get on with his job in his own way, and did so.

However, he had appreciated the need to scan Gram preparations of acutely inflamed appendices, if not on the scale that his board had asked for. He knows, now, that as many as ten per cent of these specimens may turn out to contain Grampositive, branching, finely filamentous organisms that he cannot distinguish morphologically from the pathogenic actinomycetes. Usually these organisms are sparse, and confined to the faecal contents of the lumen. He knows that this figure of ten per cent is smaller than the proportion of healthy people who have such organisms in the mouth or bowel. He knows that some of the filamentous organisms isolated from normal or inflamed appendices have the cultural characteristics of *Actinomyces israelii*. He knows also that *Actinomyces israelii* does not become even a secondary invader of anything approaching such a proportion of appendices inflamed through other causes.

The pathologist also knows, and knew long before the events of this history, that *Actinomyces israelii* is occasionally the cause of appendicitis. But this is in a fraction of one per cent of cases. He will not diagnose actinomycotic appendicitis unless he is able to demonstrate the organism actually within the wall of the appendix: its presence merely in exudate in the lumen has no recognizable pathogenic significance. In fact, because of the frequency of such organisms in the bowel contents, he never feels very confident about the diagnosis of actinomycosis unless there are well-formed colonial granules in the purulent exudate in the tissues. Such colonies are unlikely to be present unless the infection is of longer standing than is consistent with a history typical of acute appendicitis. Nevertheless, the diagnosis of actinomycotic appendicitis has sometimes to be made in their absence. Because of the long period of treatment—months—that this diagnosis generally demands, it is a diagnosis requiring exceptional consideration.

Postscript. Through over-preference for equating the pathogenic significance of actinomycetes in the appendix with their formation of colonial granules, the pathologist has just (1971) been nearly self-persuaded into interpreting as pathogenically insignificant the presence of short, fine, Gram-positive filaments that turned out to be *Nocardia asteroides*, an actinomycete that does not ordinarily form granules in the tissues. This is the first time that he has come across nocardial appendicitis, in practice and in the literature:

> The patient, a girl of 14, developed nocardial peritonitis immediately after appendicectomy. Nocardial septicaemia and nocardial meningitis followed. She was treated with sulphadiazine sodium and ampicillin, and recovered.
>
> Five days before the acute onset of clinically typical acute appendicitis, she had had a suction abortion as a hospital out-patient. An impacted wisdom tooth had been drawn while she was still under the anaesthetic. A relation between these operations and the development of nocardiosis is unproved. There was no evidence that either was followed by any form of local sepsis. *Nocardia asteroides* is an occasional constituent of the normal flora of the airways, mouth and bowel. I do not know of its isolation from the genital tract in either sex.

Appendix 1

Extracts from the pathologist's memorandum to his hospital management board on conditionally accepting the board's directive on the need and means to recognize actinomyces in the appendix:

The records of the laboratory over the last ten years show that it has received on average five acutely inflamed appendices every two weeks—130 a year.

The average acutely inflamed appendix, fixed in formalin, measures 6 cm in length and 0·9 cm in mean diameter.

Assuming that paraffin sections of surgical specimens are usually 10 microns thick (and most laboratories would expect to cut them at least 2 microns less than this), each millimetre of an embedded block of tissue provides 100 sections.

There is a choice between a technically ideal and a less satisfactory but more economical procedure for preparing the appendix for sectioning, 'Procedure A' and 'Procedure B'.

Procedure A: The appendix is serially sectioned transversely from apex to base. For the appendix of average length (6 cm) the product would be 6000 sections.

Procedure B: The appendix is divided into two equal lengths (2 × 3 cm), each of which is embedded and then sectioned not transversely but lengthwise. For the appendix of average diameter (0·9 cm) the product would be 1800 sections (900 from each of two blocks). However, this would provide diagnostically less acceptable sections, for the transverse plane is indisputably the better for examining changes in a structure such as the vermiform appendix.

Economy, both of resources and of man-hours, demands that the specimen be sectioned so that its entirety may be serialized in the smallest number of sections. This means adopting 'Procedure B'— 1800 sections for the average acutely inflamed appendix.

The Board's directive stipulates that alternate sections be stained by different methods. The only practical way to do this is to mount the sections individually, one to a slide, alternate slides being separated to form two batches. Each batch can then be subjected to bulk staining.*

* What a lot of time and effort would have been savable, by the technicians preparing the material and by the pathologists examining it, if the board had required staining alternate ribbons of serial sections, not alternate sections, by the two methods. It would then have been practicable to mount alternate ribbons on glass plates of up to, say, the common photographic 8·3 × 10·8 cm format, which is about the largest size that can be handled conveniently on a microscope stage. Such plates can easily carry 63 cross sections of an appendix or 18 longitudinal sections each 3 cm long. About a hundred plates would carry the whole appendix, whether cut transversely or lengthwise. Unfortunately, cover-glasses of this size, when obtainable, are very expensive. The development of alterna-

This procedure will make necessary the preparation of at least 1800 separately numbered standard microscope slides. This is a formidable task. Each slide will have to be indelibly marked with the laboratory number of the specimen, the number of the paraffin block and the number of the serial section—an average of twelve marks, including the necessary separators between the different numbers. For example, 'A24/59–2–117'—the 117th serial section from the 2nd paraffin block of the 24th appendix examined in 1959.

Cutting, mounting, staining and covering 1800 serial sections singly is difficult to translate into technician-hours. These operations alone might be expected to occupy the full time of a trained and skilled technician for at least four days, and possibly double that. Assuming four days to be a reasonable estimate, the five appendices received in the laboratory every fortnight would require twenty days' work, or the services of two senior technicians working a five-day week, with two juniors to assist and for contingencies (sickness, holidays and continuity).

As it would be irresponsibly wasteful to employ a pathologist to examine so large a number of sections for the presence of actinomycetes, consideration should be given to training a cadre of special screeners to do this work under supervision and report any suspect structures to the duty epityphlopathologist.* How such

---

tive methods of covering the stained sections on such plates would require a substantial investment in research. The preparations should be durable, so that they may be stored for an indefinite period in case clinical developments at any time necessitate review. Further, the plates carrying the Gram-stained sections would have to be manufactured to specifications of uniform flatness and thickness that would enable the preparations to be examined under the × 100 oil immersion objective when mounted under a coverglass (or suitable substitute). The × 100 objective has a limited working distance and cannot be used if the combined depth of mounting medium and cover exceeds this. Experience has shown that objectives of less magnifying power are not reliable when the search is for very sparse, bacillus-like filamentous forms of actinomycetes, even when contrastingly stained by a Gram method.

The board, however, by its insistence on alternate sections being differently processed, had made such considerations as these merely theoretical.

* The use of this specialist designation in the pathologist's memorandum resulted in an allegation by a member of the management that the document, far from being a serious and in intention helpful statement, was a deliberately disrespectful impertinence that raised the gravest doubts of the pathologist's qualification to hold his consultant appointment, even in an honorary capacity. Looked at impartially, the document was without doubt an impertinence, but equally its intention seems to have been helpful, and in the event its effect was helpful in that the pathologist was able to continue to provide an effective service that was neither unsafe nor extravagant.

potential screeners might be recruited and the terms and conditions of their employment are matters not within the immediate competence of this document.

Appendix 2

Gram's stain. Some contemporary views: please refer to page 28.

Reference

(1)   Symmers, W. St C. (1967) Curiosa et exotica—a selection of clinicopathological observations of unusual presentations and manifestations of familiar diseases (Case 1). *Journal of Postgraduate Medicine, 13* (October), 143–50.

6   Anti-Antigram

A medical student, having just finished her preclinical studies, spent two weeks of her vacation working as an orderly in the casualty department of the county hospital in the English town where she lived. On her last day in the department she had to hold a young gipsy while the doctor on duty took a throat swab. The boy had been brought by his mother because he had a sore throat and his breath smelt.

The doctor, who spoke English badly, was uncommunicative. He ignored the student, apart from accepting her assistance. The nurses were antagonistic to an amateur working in the hospital without pay: the student found it diplomatic not to bother them with questions—she learnt much by her own quiet observation. She noted that the doctor ordered an injection of penicillin for the child and also a dose of serum: she did not catch the name of the latter and she could not decipher what the staff nurse wrote in the treatment book.

While she held the child, the doctor's manipulation of the swab made him retch and cough—something smeared her glasses and she felt a small splash in one eye. The doctor glanced at her impatiently, but said nothing. After seeing the child into the ambulance that was to take him to the fever hospital, she cleaned her glasses and looked at her eyes—she saw no trace of what had splashed her. She washed her face and, for the time, forgot the incident. Next day she left for a month's motoring in northern Scandinavia.

Half way through the tour, the eye that had been splashed became itchy, red and swollen. There was a little yellow discharge from the conjunctiva and a lot of crusting of the lids. Bathing with water did no good. The inflammation quickly became severe and painful. Her father took her to the local doctor—the only doctor in scores of miles of scantily populated, barren countryside. The family's few words of Scandinavian languages and the doctor's smattering of English were together enough for him to follow the girl's story.

The doctor swabbed the inside of the lower eyelid, made a film of the exudate on a microscope slide and stained it by a Gram method. He produced a beautifully kept microscope, an instrument of lacquered brass, fully two feet tall, a collectors' piece, obviously still much cherished in use. The girl had never seen its like, and had not known that such magnificent microscopes had existed until something similar, of comparably massive dimensions and primitive binocular design, had caught her attention when used briefly by Dr Cruickshank in an episode from *Dr Finlay's Casebook*.*

The doctor asked her to look down the microscope. He

* The BBC's series of films based on Dr A. J. Cronin's sketches of general practice in Tannochbrae between the two world wars.

made a little drawing of rod–like forms beside which he wrote 'BKL'.* She had never seen a bacteriological preparation before, but she took the little rods to be bacteria: the doctor nodded his approval when she said so. He gave her an injection of diphtheria antitoxin (it was an English product and she took the opportunity to read the label). He also gave her an injection of penicillin and a penicillin eye ointment. In a few days the inflammation had disappeared. She had no further symptoms, except that during the next week the somewhat alarming experience of seeing double on looking to the affected side and of some difficulty in close reading caused a passing worry.

When the student got home, her family doctor asked the hospital about the gipsy boy and found that the diagnosis of diphtheria had been confirmed bacteriologically. It may hardly be doubted that the child's reflex cough had infected the girl's eye and that her conjunctivitis was diphtherial. She had never been immunized against diphtheria.

Comment

This Scandinavian doctor, working unassisted to provide a comprehensive service to a scattered community in tough country, is his own laboratory technician and pathologist, radiographer and radiologist, anaesthetist and surgeon, midwife and obstetrician. He showed himself ready as a matter of course to use Gram's stain as a means of diagnosis. He may be surprised that across the sea, in a land where some of his countrymen still train for his profession, there are responsible teachers whose influential scorn for those traditional aspects of teaching that they think valueless threatens to remove such

---

* Bacillus Klebs-Löffler, no doubt. 'KLB' to us . . . or on formal occasions *Corynebacterium diphtheriae*.

simple laboratory procedures from the experience of medical students:

> 'There's no point in expecting students to know how to do Gram's stain.'
> 'For one thing, it's difficult to do properly. For another, they'll never have occasion to use it.'
> 'And if they did, they wouldn't have a microscope anyway.'
> 'Anyway, what are laboratories for? Do we really want doctors in their surgeries to dabble, more or less incompetently, certainly without experience, in work that is best done by trained technicians in proper laboratories under controlled conditions?'

The argument is easier to put than to rebut. It is an argument of some sincere reformers of the curriculum, particularly of some teachers in pathology whose orientation is to the scientific basis of their subject rather than to its applications in practice.

'Are we training technicians or scientists?'—the question was put rhetorically by a reforming pathologist. It begs another: *'Are we training scientists or doctors?'* As it stands, neither question is creditable.

Is Gram Staining Really Necessary?

It is, of course. The case does not have to be argued here: instead, a note may be made of some cases in which Gram staining was the key to the diagnosis. In the cases of actinobacillosis on page 1 and staphylococcal infection on page 6, it was because Gram preparations were made that the organisms were distinguished from actinomyces: the distinction made, wrong and potentially dangerous treatment was avoided. In another case of actinosimulation (page 12), a Gram stain on the biopsy material would surely have prevented the misdiagnosis that occurred. It may be true that in such cases the correct diagnosis might be expected to result from other eventual investigations, in the absence of Gram staining: the fact remains that in some it *is* Gram staining that indicates the nature of the condition, and that in the circumstances of individual cases the true diagnosis might be overlooked but for this.

Question: Name any one condition in which from your own experience you would expect Gram staining to facilitate the diagnosis to such an extent that, but for this investigation, the true nature of the infection would frequently go unrecognized, with consequent hazard to the patient. Briefly state the case for your views.

Answer: Infection by *Nocardia asteroides*—Gram's stain selectively shows this Gram-positive, filamentous, often bacillus-like actinomycete in very clear contrast to the counterstained background of pus. The organism is easily overlooked in films of exudate or sections of infected tissues when these are stained by non-selective methods. The organism is also acid-fast, and in Ziehl–Neelsen preparations is liable to be taken for the tubercle bacillus unless Gram preparations are also examined. Its acid-fastness does not always withstand the processing of the tissues in the preparation of paraffin sections: ZN staining may therefore fail to show it in the latter. Again, as the exudate in nocardiosis is purulent, a ZN stain may be thought unnecessary as pus formation is so rarely a feature of tuberculosis.

The diagnosis of actinomycosis also is facilitated by Gram staining. This is important in those cases in which colonial 'grains' have not yet formed.* In such circumstances Gram staining is particularly important, for reasons similar to those

---

* See the case of the expensive appendix, page 15.

mentioned above in relation to infection by *Nocardia asteroides*. Being anaerobic or micro-aerophilic, *Actinomyces israelii* may be missed on culturing infected material unless the need for the appropriate investigations has been foreseen: again, it is in such circumstances that Gram staining may be the key to the diagnosis.

7   *Appendicitis*

We seem to be involved for the moment in a succession of the adventures and misadventures of patients (and their doctors) in hospital. Here is another that started with appendicitis.

A previously healthy young man was admitted to hospital in 1943 with uncomplicated acute appendicitis. The complications were to follow. The appendix was removed and convalescence was without incident until the day of his discharge from the ward, ten days after the operation, when he complained of pains in the chest. These were considered to be 'neurotic' and, as it had been arranged, so he was sent home. That night he was readmitted, with multiple pulmonary infarcts, the result of embolism after thrombosis of the deep veins in the calves.

There was no evidence of further embolism after his return to hospital. The infarcts gradually disappeared and he was left with no signs of interference with pulmonary function or circulation. The day came, some six weeks after the initial infarction, when he was again due to go home. That morning he complained of 'tightness' in the throat. He was firmly but kindly told that this time he really was being neurotic and, as it had been arranged, so he was sent home. That night he was seen by his family doctor, who forthwith packed him off to the fever hospital with diphtheria.

He was given antitoxic serum and responded quickly. Swabs confirmed the clinical diagnosis. There was considerable medical and administrative activity in the general hospital to trace the source of his infection (unsuccessful) and to prevent an outbreak (successful).

Following his treatment for diphtheria, every third convalescent throat swab grew pathogenic diphtheria bacilli. This continued with unbroken regularity throughout the next eight months, during which he was wholly free from symptoms and bored to distraction by incarceration as the sole occupant of the diphtheria pavilion, where he was allowed no visitors (not so much because of his carrier state as because there was a war on and civilians were excluded from the area). Eventually, ten months after developing acute appendicitis, a run of three negative throat swabs allowed his return to home and work, safe and apparently sound.

8 'The Appendix was Removed through a Neat Small Incision'

A 20-year-old woman student was admitted to a hospital's observation ward after a motor-car accident. She had been unconscious for a few minutes after striking her head against the windscreen and was still dazed when brought to the hospital half an hour later. A few hours after admission she vomited and complained of increasing headache and a bruised feeling in her abdomen. She said that she had felt sick earlier on the day of the accident, before it happened, and that she had occasionally had similar abdominal discomfort before. She was menstruating but she said that her periods did not cause pain or sickness.

The house surgeon was worried that the symptoms might be from an intracranial injury. He found no abnormality in the patient's abdomen except slight tenderness in the right iliac fossa. There was a hardly visible linear scar, four centimetres long and about four centimetres medial to the right anterior superior iliac spine: she explained that her appendix had been removed three years earlier because of chronic appendicitis. The houseman made some remark about the neatness of the scar and the patient then mentioned that the operation had been done by Mr ———, a surgeon in the city where she had been at school, and that the scar ought to be neat as he had charged her father eighty guineas for the operation (a respectable fee in the 1930s).

32

The patient continued to complain of headache and sickness, and became drowsy. Her pulse rate and temperature were rising and she had a leucocytosis. The house surgeon was very much concerned. There seemed nothing clearly pointing to an abdominal emergency, though there was some greater discomfort on palpation of the right iliac fossa than before. He found no evidence of rising intracranial pressure. He telephoned his chief again and went through the whole history with him, in more detail than before. When he mentioned the name of the surgeon who had done the appendicectomy his chief reacted at once: 'Why didn't you say so before? ——— operated? Three years ago? Right! We must open her —she probably does have an acute appendix.'

The laparotomy confirmed this. The acutely inflamed appendix, near to bursting, was removed. Convalescence was straightforward. The patient's only eventual complaint was that the scar of her second appendicectomy was bigger and more conspicuous than the first one. But it cost nothing.

Background. Mr ——— was known for his smoothness as an operator. The neatness of his incision accounted for part of his success with his patients. His cut for an interval appendicectomy was never more than four centimetres, and always delicately closed by a subcuticular stitch so that not so much as the mark of a stay suture blemished the usually almost invisible end-result.

He was an advocate of prophylactic appendicectomy, expressing the view that removal of an appendix while it was still normal would prevent acute appendicitis and an unsightly scar, or worse. His younger women patients, many of them from well-to-do families, were sometimes scandalously rumoured to be interested in the then new and hardly proper fashion for two-piece bathing costumes: why this should have boosted a demand for his services as appendicectomist is not clear, for the relevant half of such apparel in those days was more than adequate to cover completely a scar thrice the length of those that he left.

One day, it was let out by a dismissed member of the nursing staff of a private hospital where he often operated that, sometimes at least, the beautiful incision was no more than skin deep. Understandably little attention was paid to this incredible slander, at least at first, though some of his colleagues felt that in the general interests of both professions he ought to take action to clear his name and expose his detractor. He replied that to do this would itself not accord with the best traditions of Medicine: indeed, it was said that he was so generous-hearted, even to those who hurt him, that he had quietly made it possible for the unfortunate woman to emigrate and set herself up in private nursing in a far land.

Not long afterwards, the quick succession in another city of two near fatal cases of peritonitis from rupture of the acutely inflamed appendix, not diagnosed in time because the surgeons had been misled by the history of appendicectomy by Mr——— previously, confirmed the story that had been put round. The pressure that was then put on Mr ——— by his colleagues was such that he reverted to the less conservative operation.

Footnote. After operating on the patient whose later history has been told here, Mr ——— had written to her family doctor, describing her case and what he had found it necessary to do for her. His letter ended with the line 'The appendix was removed through a neat small incision'. It is the GP's amendment to this note, three years later, that accounts for the title of this chapter.

9 The Specialist

A gynaecologist removed an ovarian dermoid from a young woman. The tumour, of moderate size and on the right side, had been found when the patient was seen because of occasional attacks of vague lower abdominal pain, mainly on the right. She was chesty after the operation, and coughing caused her a good deal of pain in the region of the wound. On the fifth morning her temperature went up to 39° centigrade, her pulse was fast and she had a neutrophil leucocytosis. The abdomen was distended, and there was tenderness, particularly in the right lower quadrant.

Suspecting some local complication of the ovarian operation, the gynaecologist reopened the abdomen. He found early peritonitis from perforation of the appendix, which was gangrenous. He sent for a general surgeon who took over and removed the appendix. The patient's convalescence from that time was straightforward.

The gynaecologist explained that, although he had noticed at the time of the ovariotomy that the appendix was fibrotic and probably contained a faecolith, he did not take it out because he considered it wrong to meddle in the province of general surgery.

10   The Generalist

A general surgeon was called to see a young housewife who was a patient in a gynaecological ward and had collapsed with vomiting and sudden, severe abdominal pain during a bimanual examination. She had been admitted for investigation of irregularity of her periods, dating from her marriage a few months before. The junior gynaecologist who was examining her when she collapsed had a reputation among some of his contemporaries for being ungentle and ungentlemanly with hospital patients. His chiefs saw only his technical ability and a flattering charm that they did not seem to know was largely reserved for those with favours in their pocket. They cannot have been aware of the earthiness that distressed or outraged many of his patients and brought him the contempt of the nursing staff and the dislike of many of his medical colleagues.

The patient, formerly an assistant on the administrative staff of the hospital and aware of the gynaecologist's reputation, had looked forward with growing anxiety and tenseness to being examined by him. A good year earlier she had been under medical treatment for a radiologically proved duodenal ulcer: when she collapsed the gynaecologist assumed that her ulcer had perforated. The general surgeon agreed, and opened her abdomen—it was full of blood from a ruptured tubal pregnancy. He sent at once for the gynaecologist, who had left for another hospital, but returned and within twenty minutes of his colleague's call for help had stopped the bleeding and removed the tube. Until the specialist arrived the

36

general surgeon had held a swab against the bleeding area, in a not very effectual effort to control the blood loss. The delay in dealing with the emergency nearly cost the patient her life, for she was bleeding much more than the surgeon realized and was almost exsanguinated.

The general surgeon explained that he had not dealt with the tubal rupture himself because, although he had assisted at such operations while a student and was familiar with the procedure, he did not consider it right to meddle in the province of a specialty.

11 Red Tape

The wife of a doctor found a small lump in one breast. She and her husband thought this unlikely to be malignant, but they consulted a surgeon with a view to having it removed and examined in the laboratory. The surgeon thought it likely to be benign. It came as a surprise to him, and as a shock to his patient and her husband, when the pathologist regarded the appearances in the frozen sections as equivocal. When the paraffin sections came through next day three senior pathologists saw them and disagreed on the interpretation: the head of the department felt certain that the lesion was benign—not a tumour at all, in fact, but a somewhat unusual form of fibrosing adenosis (Figs 11.1 and 11.2); his two younger colleagues were convinced that it was an adenocarcinoma. Because, with good reason, the younger men respected their chief's histological acumen, they thought it would be foolish for the surgeon to do a radical operation on the grounds of their interpretation alone.

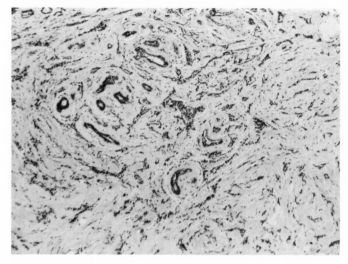

Fig. 11.1.   Although at first sight it would seem that this field was from a somewhat scirrhous mammary adenocarcinoma, it is in fact a benign state—a form of fibrosing adenosis. No one used to reporting on rapid frozen sections will have any trouble in appreciating that this specimen was a potentially equivocal one. There was no discredit in the fact that three experienced histopathologists found themselves in disagreement over the diagnosis, two to one. Nor is it discreditable that on this occasion it was the opinion of the majority that was wrong.

Cryostat section; haematoxylin–eosin   × 75

The surgeon agreed that diagnostic arbitration should be sought elsewhere. A certain honest humility kept him from influencing his laboratory colleagues by voicing his impression that what he saw down the microscope was hyperplastic, within the limits of his experience, not cancerous. Characteristically, he under-rated those limits. Yet his own histological impression may at least have strengthened his belief that a delay before the diagnosis was settled would not endanger the patient. It was decided to send sections to a pathologist in another country.

The neat little parcel of slides was posted in the air mail box at the General Post Office, appropriately marked for special

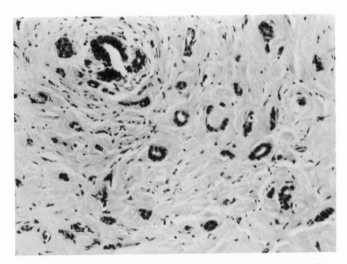

Fig. 11.2.   In the isolated field, higher magnification does not necessarily at once resolve the problem of interpretation illustrated in Fig. 11.1. Here, for instance, it is no easier to recognize the benign nature of this lesion than at the lower power of the microscope, for now the picture might be thought to be that of a well-differentiated scirrhous adenocarcinoma. Yet what might seem carcinomatous tubules are atrophic acini and ducts in a lobule that has undergone fibrosis following a hyperplastic phase.

Paraffin section; haematoxylin–eosin   × 130

delivery in the city of its destination, and labelled 'VERY URGENT—PATHOLOGICAL SLIDES FOR DIAGNOSIS—NOT DANGEROUS—NO COMMERCIAL VALUE'. Unfortunately, the usually meticulous clerk who posted it miscalculated the cost of the air mail charges and the special delivery fee: he understamped the package by eight cents, a tiny proportion of the correct total cost. That was on a Wednesday afternoon, the day after the operation on the patient. On the Friday of that week the parcel was returned by the GPO for the lacking eight cents to be added in further stamps, so that the addressee might be saved the inconvenience of having to pay a postage-due fee.

Unluckily, the returned parcel was not delivered to the pathology department but to the general office of the hospital.

The hospital had a regulation that, through need for economy, no parcels might be sent by air mail unless this had been specially authorized by a senior member of the administrative staff. This regulation was regularly disregarded by the clinical departments, most of which dispatched their mail themselves, paying for it out of their petty cash accounts. It was not until Monday of the next week, six days after the operation on the patient, that the parcel was seen by the appropriately senior administrator, who at once authorized the additional expenditure of eight cents. Next day it was posted again. Its twelve thousand miles journey was quickly completed, it was not delayed in the customs offices, and on the afternoon of Maundy Thursday the post office delivered it by special messenger.

The parcel was addressed to the pathologist, by name, at the pathology department of the medical school where he worked. It happened to be the case that, by longstanding agreement, all post sent to departments or individuals at any of the school's addresses was delivered to the school office, in a commercial block only a short way from the buildings that housed the various departments. Ordinarily, this arrangement worked satisfactorily enough. But on Maundy Thursday, in anticipation of the Easter holiday weekend, the school office had closed early. When the postal messenger arrived there was no one there but a cleaner, who accepted the little parcel and put it in the box for incoming mail. There it was found on the next Wednesday, when the office opened after the holiday. The pathologist received it that morning, eight days after it finally left the hospital oversea and fifteen days after the operation on the patient. The laboratory staff, continuing throughout the holiday to deal with their hospital's biopsy specimens, had no way of knowing that an urgent specimen, arrived by post from oversea, was waiting in the administrative offices down the street.

By the time the pathologist had looked again at the sections, thought about them, discussed them with others in the department, and concluded that he could give a reasonably confident opinion, it was four o'clock in his afternoon and one o'clock in the morning of the next day where the patient was. He therefore decided not to telephone his distant colleague, for it seemed that a telegram by the fastest route would be as effectively prompt in carrying his view that the lesion was benign.

Unknown to the pathologist, his secretary had not been able to pass the telegram to the cable office herself, because of a new standing order in the hospital, which shared its telephone switchboard with the school. This order, which in the occasional nature of such things had not been made known to the school, laid down that no telegrams might be sent without the authorization of a senior member of the hospital's administrative staff. The pathologist's secretary, therefore, had had to dictate the telegram to a switchboard operator at the hospital, but assumed that it would be sent without delay. The switchboard operator referred the telegram to the administrative officer for authorization. The administrator was at a committee meeting when the text of the telegram was put on his desk: he did not see it until late in the afternoon of the next day, Thursday. He immediately authorized its dispatch and on the Friday morning his secretary handed it to the switchboard staff, who immediately telephoned it to the cable office.

The telegram arrived at its destination after the working day, on Friday, was over. It was taken by hand from the hospital's reception desk to the pathology department and there left in the office in-tray, where it was found on Monday morning and at once handed to the pathologist. As he read it, one of his colleagues was in the biopsy room, dissecting the radical mastectomy specimen, removed from the patient on the day before, Sunday, nineteen days after the first operation.

Later on that Monday, the local telegraph company got in touch with the pathologist who had waited so long in vain for an answer to his original biopsy problem. They reported that the telegram that he had sent five days earlier, to hasten a reply from his colleague, had been returned to the office of its origin because the address was insufficient for delivery. In fact, the address was wrong in only one respect—a laboratory clerk had written New York instead of London, her mind being on other things. It was because there had been no reply to this telegram that the decision had been taken to act on the local majority opinion and do the radical operation.

Footnote. There was no evidence of a tumour in the mastectomy specimen.

Advice to a Consultant. Another time—when you've made up your mind, telephone the result, then, yourself.*

* *Question*: Even after midnight?

12 A Mastectomy for No Good Reason . . .[1]

This is a history that I had not meant to include among these *Curiosa* and *Exotica*, but the patient and her husband—he was the surgeon who operated on her—have asked that it be told again. They had heard of *Curiosa* at a supper party in the home of colleagues. One of the other guests amused the mainly medical company with readings from the draft typescript, which had been sent to him in confidence by a publisher's reader who wanted advice on whether to accept it.

The couple, anxious to save others from such an experience as they had, feel that their inclusion complements some of the other histories in these pages.

History. It all happened quite a long time ago. The patient, working in hospital, was accidentally jabbed in the right breast with a needle that had just been used in aspirating pus from a child's subperiosteal abscess. An acute abscess followed the injury. Several millilitres of pus were evacuated through a stab incision about half a centimetre long: the cavity in the breast was filled with a then much used proprietary paste of bismuth and iodoform in liquid paraffin, and the wound was covered with an occlusive dressing. *Staphylococcus aureus* was grown from the pus. When the dressing was removed, a week later, the incision had healed though the underlying tissues remained indurated.

Two months later, a slightly tender, nodular mass, a couple of centimetres across, was felt at the site, fixed to the skin and to the pectoral muscle. The mass grew slowly. After another

43

month there was dimpling over it and a *'peau d'orange'* appearance. A cluster of lymph nodes had become palpable under the anterior axillary fold.

The surgeon took the lesion for a chronic staphylococcal granuloma, though he was concerned to note the changes in the skin that could indicate the presence instead of a carcinoma. Attempts at aspiration yielded nothing, so he excised the affected part. When, immediately after its removal, he bisected the mass he found it to be hard, solid, and speckled with small yellow spots from which thin coils of cheese-like matter appeared when the tissue was squeezed. From the macroscopical appearances he diagnosed the lesion as a 'comedo cancer' with scirrhous change.* He was certain enough of the significance of the naked eye appearances not to ask for a frozen section—at that time a rare procedure, grudgingly undertaken and of correspondingly limited reliability. With no more ado he performed a radical mastectomy.

Microscopical examination showed that the mass was a sclerosing oleogranuloma (Fig. 12.1). Oleogranulomatous foci were also present in the nearer axillary lymph nodes. There was no sign of any neoplasm. The cheesy material was shown to contain liquid paraffin and bismuth—it was the remains of the paste that had been packed into the abscess cavity three months before.

Comment

There is no doubt that it was the liquid paraffin that caused the granuloma. Individuals seem to vary considerably in the extent, speed and severity of their reaction to this material, which is only one of a variety of 'oily' substances that can

---

* In other words, a scirrhous infiltrating carcinoma arising from and overgrowing intraduct carcinoma. Necrotic tumour at the core of the intraduct growth can be expressed from the cut surface in a fashion likened to an acne comedo squeezed from its follicle.

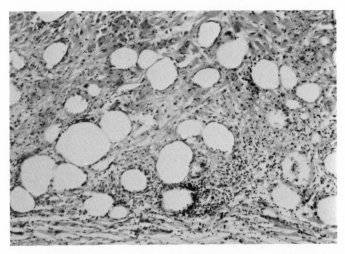

Fig. 12.1.   Sclerosing oleogranuloma. The larger of the apparently clear spaces contained liquid paraffin that has disappeared in the process of histological preparation. There are many large, opaque macrophages in the intervening tissue, a finding that sometimes leads to misinterpretation of such lesions as 'granular cell myoblastoma', perhaps particularly in the breast, which is one of the sites where the latter is recognized to occur.

Haematoxylin–eosin   × 70

cause troublesome or dangerous granulomas when introduced into the tissues.

When this story was published in 1955, with five more or less comparable other cases of oil granulomas simulating cancers, the histories were selected out of a series of fourteen similar observations provided by colleagues at home and oversea.[1] The fifteen and more years since then have brought in as many more such cases: fortunately, the proportion in which the real nature of the lesion was recognized before any radical surgery has been far higher than in the original series. Awareness of the condition and more use of biopsy, including frozen sections, have had this effect.

Oleogranuloma is still to be reckoned with in clinical diagnosis.

Reference

(1) Symmers, W. St C. (1955) Simulation of cancer by oil granulomas of therapeutic origin. *British Medical Journal, 2* (December 24), 1536–9.

13 . . . Another Mastectomy for No Good Reason . . .

A distinguished scientist was appointed to succeed a distinguished practising pathologist as head of a university department. He was chosen for his international reputation in a specialized field of non-clinical research. His new duties required that he accept nominal responsibility for diagnostic work that the department undertook for local hospitals and practitioners on a contractual basis. The service was already well organized and efficient, and he had merely to allow the work to be carried out by the specialist staff employed for the purpose: in exchange, he was himself given a contract that would entitle him to a substantial and regular financial reward above his salary in return for the 'clinical responsibilities' that he accepted in this *ex officio* capacity. It was many years since he had done any diagnostic laboratory work, and he was glad that in practice his new job would not make it necessary for him to revert.

Things went smoothly for some years. Then, one day, the concurrence of epidemic influenza, acute appendicitis, an international congress and a temporarily disabling road accident left the histopathology laboratory with only a trainee pathologist in attendance. The trainee dealt competently with the straightforward reporting, by day: in the evenings he was able to take all the day's sections that he was not sure about to the freshly appendicectomized consultant, who had had a microscope installed on his bed-table to lessen the tedium of convalescence. The head of the department felt that he could contribute nothing except moral support for the trainee: he was not worried about the shortage of staff—the congress that had deprived the department of the services of two members would not last long, and two more would at any moment be back from their brief capitulation to the 'flu virus.

Then the unforeseen happened, foreseeably. A senior surgeon in the town—a blunt, irascible man, and uncompromisingly critical of the faculty's policy in appointing a 'research man' to run a once traditional department of pathology—was asked to see the 21-year-old eldest daughter of an influential local family. She had a clinically equivocal lump in a breast. Unaware of the depleted state of the department's diagnostic staff, the surgeon sent the freshly excised specimen for an immediate frozen section. He regarded himself as senior enough not to need to send word to the laboratory of the likelihood of such an examination being required in the course of any of his operating sessions. The additional delay caused by this misconception regularly amplified his impatience as, on each such occasion, he stood by the anaesthetized patient, waiting for the result before being able to decide how to complete the operation.

This time, when the tumour arrived unheralded in the laboratory, the trainee, on his own, had no choice but to send word to the surgeon that he was alone and without experience to report safely on a frozen section. The surgeon, perhaps the more enraged for realizing his fault in not getting in touch with the laboratory beforehand, angrily demanded an immediate opinion on the sections from the head of the department, who, incapable of resisting a bully, gave in. As a young man the head had worked for a time in a laboratory that dealt with biopsies and PMs among the general run of a service in clinical pathology. Maybe those days were some justification for avoiding the embarrassment that refusing the surgeon's demand would have brought. Moreover, though he had not had occasion to deal with human tissues for many years, his own work had made him familiar with the microscopical appearances of various natural and experimental diseases of small laboratory animals.

The scientist looked at the frozen section. What he saw seemed, he thought, to resemble a mammary carcinoma that he was acquainted with in a strain of mice. The impression of familiarity restored some of his confidence: he reported the section as showing 'epithelial proliferation and disorganization of pattern not altogether inconsistent with carcinoma'.

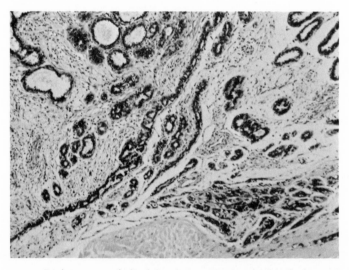

Fig. 13.1.   Both stroma and glandular elements are involved in the hyperplasia. This field shows how compression of epithelial tissue between adjoining foci of stromal proliferation produces the fibroadenomatoid pattern. It is in such areas of compression that the picture may be mistaken for carcinomatous infiltration. The distinction from carcinoma is particularly difficult in frozen sections, and there are cases in which it cannot then be made. See Fig. 13.2 also (and Figs 41.2 and 42.1, pages 179 and 178).

Haematoxylin–eosin   × 70

It was the last word of the report that registered with the surgeon. He was accustomed to teaching that the clinician must be able to reduce laboratory reports to essentials, and the 'essential' in this frozen section report was 'carcinoma'. He was disappointed rather than surprised that this was the finding—after all, it had been because there was some room for clinical doubt that he had needed the frozen section at all, and now the outcome confirmed his good sense in entertaining the possibility that his clinical intuition could be at fault . . . He did a radical mastectomy.

The regular histopathologists returned to the department on the next day. They saw the sections of the tumour and

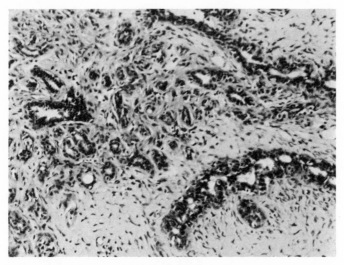

Fig. 13.2.   This is the sort of area that may invite interpretation as adenocarcinomatous yet is in fact part of the hyperplastic state. The distinction is subjective and learnt by frequent and long experience—to try to put its many bases into words continues to defeat the writers of texts, and within the limits of our present histological knowledge and methods there will always be that small proportion of cases in which even the best authorities differ in their diagnosis. That conflict would hardly develop over the findings in the case in this chapter, which were nowhere more difficult to interpret than in these representative fields.

Haematoxylin–eosin   × 120

that it was a simple, typical focus of fibroadenomatoid hyperplasia, wholly benign (Figs 13.1 and 13.2). And when they examined the mastectomy specimen it too showed no sign of any neoplastic disease.

Aftermath. Shocked by what he considered her mutilation, the patient's fiancé broke his engagement. She has not married.

Sequel. The head of the pathology department survived the surgeons' efforts to have him unseated. He asked and won their support for a reorganization of responsibilities in the department, with practising pathologists in full charge of the diagnostic laboratories.

14 . . . and Likewise an Excision of Rectum[1]

A young man developed an acute abscess in the left ischiorectal fossa. The abscess was incised, the pus evacuated and the cavity packed with gauze tape that had been smeared thickly with yellow soft paraffin in order to make its eventual withdrawal easier. During the following week the packing was extracted, a few centimetres at a time, until by the eighth day its removal was completed.

A month later there was still a small discharging sinus at the site of the incision. A firm mass, fixed to the mucosa, could be felt through the rectal wall in the ischiorectal fossa of that side. Although nothing abnormal was seen on proctoscopy, the mass was thought to be a carcinoma that had invaded the fossa from a clinically inapparent primary growth deep in the rectal mucosa or arising from submucosal glands. The fossa was explored surgically: the naked-eye findings were considered to confirm the clinical impression of cancer, and abdominoperineal excision of the rectum and ischiorectal tissues was performed without preliminary biopsy.

The sections showed that the mass was an oleogranuloma. There was no neoplasm.

The patient became increasingly depressed. He would not believe his doctors when they told him that the operation had cured the disease permanently (there is no record that he was told the real nature of the lesion). He was advised to go abroad for a rest that should ward off an incipient nervous breakdown. He died there, a few months later, from an accidental overdose of sleeping draught. The PM showed no other abnormality, apart, of course, from what the pathologist summarized as 'status post proctectomiam'—there was no cancer.

Comment

This was a case typifying the clinical mimicry of cancer by an oleogranuloma resulting from therapeutic introduction of some oily substance into the tissues. Another instance was described in Chapter 12 (page 43). As so often in such cases, one is left regretting that there was no biopsy, for it might have prevented the needlessly radical treatment.*

An oleogranulomatous reaction may be caused by true oils, liquid and solid paraffins and waxes. Some people are likelier than others to react with the formation of a massive granuloma, and some substances are likelier than others to cause this response. It is surprising how often the history of the introduction of the foreign material is not elicited, and, when it is known, how often its significance is not recognized.

---

* I once diagnosed oleogranuloma from its typical appearances in a rectal biopsy specimen. The surgeon was not satisfied, for there was a rectal ulcer that felt and looked like a carcinoma. When he repeated the biopsy operation, this time taking tissue from the margin of the ulcer instead of from the surrounding mucosa, the coexistent carcinoma was shown. The patient had had injections for piles (the latter were probably symptomatic of the growth and their treatment in no way responsible for its development).

The usual cause of a rectal oleogranuloma that simulates cancer is treatment of haemorrhoids by injections of a sclerosing agent in an oily medium.[1] Patients are sometimes reticent about admitting to having had piles, or—remarkable as it might seem to the untreated sufferer—may even forget that they ever did so, even when other rectal symptoms develop later.

Reference

(1)   Symmers, W. St C. (1955) Simulation of cancer by oil granulomas of therapeutic origin. *British Medical Journal, 2* (December 24), 1536–9.

15   Horror Story

A surgeon regularly did a ward round every Sunday morning with the final year students at his hospital. One Sunday he stopped at the bed of a young woman whose kidney he had removed, because of stone, on the Thursday before. He asked how she felt. 'Quite well, thank you, doctor', she replied, then added, 'But not as well as I did three days after you took out my other kidney three years ago.'

It was long before the days of kidney substitutes. She died a fortnight after the nephrectomy. Her blood urea reached over a thousand milligrams per hundred millilitres. Though progressively drowsier, she stayed conscious until two days before her death.

History

On the night before the fatal nephrectomy, the house surgeon had rung up his chief for their usual discussion of the cases for the next day's operating list. The chief was disappointed to hear that of the patients who had been intended for operation only one, a man with a hernia, was still available. Family trouble had taken one woman home, another was menstruating, and a staff member who belonged to the Oxford Group had misguidedly talked a third into feeling spiritually unprepared to meet the risks of major surgery. The surgeon's disappointment was evident in his voice. The HS, who did not like people to have disappointments, tried to make amends by mentioning that a woman with a renal stone had just that evening been admitted off the waiting list. The surgeon at once said that he would do her in the place of one of the cancellations.

All the HS knew about this patient was that she had been seen by one of the assistant surgeons in the out-patients department a fortnight before. She had been referred for treatment by her panel doctor, whose letter read:

> Dear dr.
> Pat. has kiddney stone.
> R & obl.
> yrs.
> Dr ———.
> Physicn. & Srgn. M.B B.cH B.A.o.

He must have made this diagnosis from her complaint of pain in one loin and blood in the water, for—as was later learnt from the patient—he had neither examined her nor asked about her earlier history. She had only recently gone on his panel, having moved to his part of town when she married. He had not received her records from the doctor whose panel she had been on before.

Three years before, when she was first found to have kidney stones, the left kidney was not functioning and was removed. The surgeon's intention had been to readmit her after convalescence and then do a pyelolithotomy on the right side. She seemed not to have been told of this, and if her doctor got the letter about it he took no action.

When, three years later, she came back to the hospital because of the reappearance of symptoms, she did not mention that she had been a patient there before. As she had changed her name on marriage, the hospital's records department failed to uncover the fact of the previous admission. The assistant surgeon in the over-busy out-patients department, having ordered and seen the straight X-ray picture before he met the patient, merely told her that she indeed had a stone and would soon be sent for to have treatment as an in-patient. He did not take her history, and he did not examine her. The scar of the nephrectomy remained unseen.

The HS on the ward had not seen the patient when he mentioned her to his chief. No one remarked that she had not had an intravenous pyelogram (which even in those days was a standard investigation before proceeding with a nephrectomy). When the chief said that she should be put on the next day's operating list, the houseman passed the instruction to the ward sister, who was just going off duty and relayed it to the staff nurse, who was too busy to do more than tell a probationer to 'prep.' the patient for the operation. The probationer saw the old nephrectomy scar, but was too occupied in chatting with the patient about other things to ask her about it; she did not mention it to any one. She cleaned the patient's skin, painted it with iodine solution, covered the area with a sterile dressing and fixed it in place with a many-tailed bandage—all was ready for the next day's operation. Later that evening, when the HS came to examine the patient, he let the night nurses talk him out of doing so—they had no intention of removing the bandage and the dressing if they could avoid it.

On the next day, Thursday, the patient was on the operating table and draped with sterile linen before the surgeon and his assistant turned from the scrubbing basins. They did not see the scar of the first nephrectomy until the Sunday after they removed the second kidney.

16 Promiscuity Polyposis

The only surviving member of the known branches of a family that for generations had suffered from polyposis of the large bowel was advised by his doctor not to marry. He accepted this advice. When he died of the disease, eight years later, he had had three children by women whom, in accordance with what the doctor had said, he had not married. One of these children died of carcinoma of the rectum at the age of fourteen. The other two, before they also died of polyposis, married and had children. At least one of this most recent generation has already died of the disease.

Comment

Familial polyposis of the large bowel is inherited as a dominant factor. It affects the sexes equally but can be transmitted only by those affected. Symptoms usually appear in the twenties and rarely after the forties. Eventually, carcinomatous change occurs in one or more of the polyps, usually in the middle thirties, some twenty-five years below the average age at which carcinoma of the large bowel ordinarily presents.

The doctor's obvious intention to advise his patient not to father any children was genetically sound. He should have said what he meant.

17 Wild Watercress

A surgeon had been feeling off colour for several weeks. He noticed that his urine was sometimes uncommonly dark. Then, one morning, shaving, he saw that his eyes had yellowed and realized that recent slight epigastric discomfort might be something more than a trivial alimentary upset. He went to see a physician, who found a tender mass in the epigastrium.

Laparotomy showed the mass to be the enlarged left lobe of the liver, part hyperaemic, part pale and part jaundiced. Under its smooth surface it felt coarsely uneven in texture, as though there were irregular foci of infiltration within it. The rest of the liver, the gall bladder and the accessible parts of the bile ducts appeared normal. Needling the affected lobe produced bile-stained pus: this was examined immediately, but no amoebae or other organisms were seen in fresh preparations on a warm-stage microscope or in stained films. The lobe was excised. Convalescence was uncomplicated.

The lobe was riddled with abscesses involving the bile ducts. It was clear that we were dealing with a suppurative cholangiitis. Because of a previous similar experience[1] the possibility of liver fluke infestation was suspected. A search of the ducts produced a typical adult liver fluke, *Fasciola hepatica* (Fig. 17.1). Several immature flukes were also present (Fig. 17.2).

The Earlier History. On an autumn day in 1967, some seven months before the start of his obstructive symptoms, friends of the surgeon had taken him for a walk in the Avon Valley

56

in the south-west of Hampshire. In keeping up with his hosts' young children, the surgeon got ahead of the rest of the party. He came on a bed of wild watercress, and plucked and ate some, offering a share to the children—they refused it, saying it was not good to take.

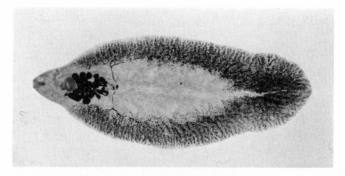

Fig. 17.1 This is the fully grown *Fasciola hepatica* that was found in one of the ducts in the excised lobe of the surgeon's liver. While the blood flukes, the schistosomes, are unisexual, the male carrying the female in his gynaecophore, the other trematodes that parasitize man—fasciola and other liver flukes, such as *Clonorchis sinensis,* and the lung fluke, *Paragonimus westermani*—are hermaphrodite. The surgeon's fluke has had its female parts injected and stained: the dense black central mass is the contorted uterus, and behind this are the fine paired vitelline ducts, coming from the vitellaria, the yolk-producing glands that are seen as the fine black stippling of the lateral and posterior parts. The male glands and ducts are not seen; they occupy mainly the central unstained region of the body. This region also accommodates the digestive system: a caecum and its lateral branches can just be made out on each side of the midline. The oral sucker is seen at the front of the fluke, forming its tip, and just in front of the injected uterus the ventral sucker can be seen as a grey ring: the parasite can attach itself to the lining of the bile duct by either sucker, but its nutriment is not drawn directly from the tissues of the host, simply being derived from the contents of the ducts that it lives in.

Cleared intact specimen, photographed by transmitted light × 3

When the children's parents caught up with the advance party they were horrified to hear what their guest had done. They were well aware of the risk of picking up fascioliasis in this way, for the infestation is prevalent in the valley of the Hampshire Avon—in places to the extent that practically all the cattle are infested and sheep cannot be raised. It had been here, in the market town of Ringwood, that the first recorded outbreak of human fascioliasis in Britain occurred, in 1958[2]: before then only a dozen or so isolated cases had been reported in these islands.

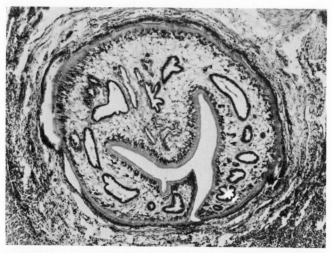

Fig. 17.2.   Cross section of an immature fasciola filling a bile duct in the lobectomy specimen. The biliary epithelium is intact at this level, as can be seen if it is followed over the surface of the fluke from the cleft between the two at the left of the field. The cuticle of the parasite has a hyaline appearance; its spines can be seen in several places, for instance from twelve to two o'clock and from six o'clock to seven. The surrounding tissues are infiltrated by leucocytes, in consequence of the severe suppurative cholangiitis that had followed obstruction of ducts by the parasites in other parts of the lobe.

Haematoxylin–eosin   × 65

The surgeon, who was not familiar with flukes, thought the whole thing a rather tiresome leg-pull. When they got home from the abruptly ended outing, his hostess gave him a one-dose bottle of piperazine elixir to take, believing (perhaps mistakenly) that it might kill any excysting metacercariae. But as soon as he got to his bedroom he poured it away.

He paid no particular attention when, a few days later, he suffered a series of short attacks of quite severe upper abdominal 'colic', with fever. Later, he remarked that it had occurred to him at the time that he might be developing cholecystitis (an idea that he had evidently been quick to dismiss as suggesting shamefully unprofessional hypochondria).

He forgot the whole episode until the pathologist came probing into his history after the lobectomy.

Comment

The usual definitive host of *Fasciola hepatica* is the sheep; other herbivorous animals are also prone to the infestation. The adult flukes live in the host's bile ducts and their ova escape in the faeces. The motile miracidia hatch from the ova and undergo encystment in the tissues of the freshwater snails (usually species of *Limnaea*) that are the intermediate hosts. About two months later the resulting cercarial form of the parasite leaves the snail and settles on waterside vegetation, becoming the metacercarial cyst, which is firmly adherent to the surface of the plant and just about visible to the naked eye as a whitish globule. The cycle continues when sheep or other animals graze by the water and swallow infested vegetation.

Human fascioliasis is rare in Britain, even in regions where the disease is prevalent in animals. We probably owe our comparative freedom from it to the fact that the only waterside plant we are at all likely to eat is the wild watercress (*Nasturtium officinale*), itself infrequent. When infested cress is eaten, the metacercariae excyst in the duodenum and make their way through the bowel wall into the peritoneal cavity. Thence, except in the rarest cases (in which they get themselves into a false position, such as the abdominal wall), they home on the liver, passing through its capsule and substance to reach the biliary passages, where they develop into mature flukes. The time between eating the infested plant and full maturation of the flukes is probably about three to four months.

There are two distinct clinical phases of human fascioliasis. First, and commoner, is the phase of invasion by the meta-cercarial larvae. The triad of acute and severe upper ab-dominal pain, enlargement of the liver and fever suggests the diagnosis: when this is accompanied by eosinophilia in the peripheral blood the syndrome is practically pathognomonic. The surgeon-patient, pertinently known for Lacedaemonian qualities of indifference to pain, admitted to no more than rather trivial effects of this phase of his infestation, already noted.

The second, or obstructive, phase develops months or years, perhaps even decades, later. The interval of seven months in the surgeon's case was uncommonly short.

A Word on Treatment. Emetine seems to be the favoured drug. It is certainly preferable to antimony compounds, such as are used in treating infestation by the blood flukes (schistoso-miasis). But no satisfactory treatment for fascioliasis has yet been found. Avoidance of the disease is therefore all the more important—and once the flukes have developed within the biliary tract they may live for very many years, while the host is constantly under the risk of developing biliary obstruc-tion and secondary bacterial infection of the ducts.

Piperazine, offered to the surgeon by his frightened hostess, is said to lessen the symptoms of invasion, though not as much as chloroquine. Chloroquine was tried in fascioliasis because of its usefulness in treating infestation by the Chinese liver fluke, *Clonorchis sinensis*. It relieves the symptoms of the invasive phase of fascioliasis: it rarely, if ever, eradicates the parasites.

Moral

Avoid wild watercress and one should escape fascioliasis.*

References

(1) Kirk, R. M. (1961) Fascioliasis presenting as a localized hepatic mass. *British Medical Journal*, 2 (November 18), 1333–4.
(2) Facey, R. V. & Marsden, P. D. (1960) Fascioliasis in man: an outbreak in Hampshire. *British Medical Journal*, 2 (August 27), 619–25.

18 Documentary

This story was told me by a television producer who works in a German-speaking part of Europe. With the object of making a documentary film, he had travelled with a group of anthropologists engaged in a field study of life in Levantine countries. There were eight in the party—five scientists (one of them a medical doctor), a cameraman, a sound recordist and the producer. They were joined by a local colleague who acted as interpreter and general way-smoother.

Having the goodwill of a mountain community, arrangements had been made to film a religious festivity that had never been recorded before. Everything was going well. The visitors were made welcome, and treated with traditional hospitality and kindness as honoured and honourable guests. Food and drink were served, and among the fare there was much that was strange to the visitors, experienced as they were in sampling all sorts of unusual provender in many parts

* I have seen wild watercress, picked in Hampshire in October by a member of the refectory staff, served as a salad at an annual dinner for the teachers at a medical school. It never appeared that anyone was any the worse, but then even the most deplorable risks are not always disastrous: that is no reason for running them.

of the world. The possibility of intestinal infections worried them little—in accordance with their contract all were taking Entero-Vioform* as a regular prophylactic against alimentary infections. Some of them, when the risks seemed great, dosed themselves with phthalylsulphathiazole or a broad-spectrum antibiotic as well.

The final course that night was served with special ceremony, shortly after a succession of animal sacrifices that were the climax of the religious devotions. This dish was clearly regarded as an exceptional delicacy. As it was put before them, their chief host spoke earnestly to the interpreter, and with an air of urgency that did not escape his guests, though they did not understand its reason from their colleague's response: he nodded his acknowledgement of the chief's words, which seemed to have caused him some momentary disquiet, then turned to the visitors. He explained that they must without fail be seen by their hosts to chew each mouthful of the delicacy—to chew fast, and strongly, and for a long time . . . This, it seemed to them, was a mandatory homage to the excellence and rarity of the food and to the unprecedented privilege of sharing it. Their colleague added, as if it were a polite consideration of their pleasure, that chewing was also necessary to ensure that the occasion should be recalled with enjoyment.

But such was the aversion caused by the look, the smell and the taste of the offering that those who did not manage to dispose covertly of their helping swallowed each inescapable mouthful as quickly as possible, before making a vigorous pretence to chew fast, strongly and long.

Within hours of the ceremony, each member of the party who had taken the special, and specially repellent, offering developed painful swelling of the throat, with blood-streaked spit. Some of them were also troubled by considerable dis-

---

* Ciba's proprietary clioquinol preparation, widely popular where intestinal infections are prevalent. Not all doctors approve of its indiscriminate use.

comfort in the ears, as if from Eustachian blockage. One developed symptoms of respiratory obstruction so alarming that the medical man felt certain he was about to have to make a tracheostomy (it turned out not to be needed).

The afflicted soon noticed that there were greyish or reddish creatures in their spit. Then they realized, with even more horror, that similar bodies were apparently attached to the lining of the throat and mouth. The creatures were flat or—especially the darker ones—rather bulbous, and not above a centimetre or so long. The flat ones were shaped something like an arrow-head; the others reminded one of the men of small leeches. In spite of their scientific training, none of the group preserved any of these bodies, which they were in no doubt were some form of parasitic animal.

Within a day or two everyone had recovered. Their local colleague, who had not been affected, seemed uncharacteristically subdued. Later, he told them that the delicacy had consisted mainly of the raw liver of freshly killed young goats,* which at that season are frequently, and often very heavily, infested by the larvae of the so-called tongue worm, *Linguatula serrata,* if not by the young of the liver fluke, *Fasciola hepatica.* Unless the parasites in the raw liver are killed by thorough chewing of each mouthful, it seems that they attach themselves to the mucous membrane of the mouth and throat, and sometimes of the nasopharynx, causing symptoms such as the group experienced. The symptoms may last no more than a few hours, though some patients are ill for several days. Death from oedema of the throat is said to have occurred, and an English milady is supposed, probably apocryphally, to have died of disgust.

* By all accounts a remarkable linguist, the local member of the party was rather less fluent in his colleagues' language than in French and English. It did nothing to lessen their disquiet when he stumbled over the German for what he knew to be *chevreau,* in French. The English equivalent—kid—came to him first, and in the embarrassment of the moment this operated the wrong circuits: '*Ihr habt alle die rohen Leber neu geopferten Kindlein gefressen*', he told them—'You have all eaten the raw livers of freshly sacrificed little children'. Their consternation quickly uncovered his error. A kid with four legs is a *Zicklein.*

The disease goes by various names, among them *halzoun,**
a vernacular word at first translated as buccopharyngeal
distomatosis and only later realized to have the alternative
meaning of buccopharyngeal pentastomiasis (larval lingua-
tuliasis). Perhaps 'parasitic pharyngitis', being an aetiologi-
cally neutral term, is preferable. It seems that, because there
has been certain proof that linguatulid larvae are responsible
for the disease,[1] the older view that immature fasciolae were
the cause has been thought to be totally instead of only in part
incorrect. The same clinical picture may be caused by each
parasite.

It is said that the linguatulid larvae first get swallowed and
then ascend the gullet to settle in the throat and even in the
mouth and nose. This sounds a likelier, if perverse, itinerary
than the simple *en passant* attachment to the mucosa during
the short time before swallowing that was the favoured
explanation of pharyngeal fasciliosis, the young flukes being
supposedly too sluggish to make their way up the oesophagus,
once swallowed, and in any case too vulnerable to peptic
digestion in the stomach to survive.

Whether they get there directly or deviously, the parasites
in the throat, mouth and nose soon fall from the mucosa and
are swallowed, either again or once and for all, according to
their identity. If they are swallowed it may be comforting to
believe that they do not, if linguatulids, live through the
second peptic exposure or, if flukes, the first. However, linguatulids that remain above the glottis are already at a stage when
all that is left for them to do to complete their life cycle is mi-
grate to the nasopharynx and nasal cavities, moult there a few
times and so become adult 'tongue worms': this occurs only
with great rarity in man, and in fact most ingested nymphs die
within a few days. It has to be added here that by no means
all young liver flukes are killed by the gastric secretions: but

---

* *Halzoun,* an Arabic word, also means snail, but in the context this does not help much
toward determining which parasites are the cause.

those that live have no future, for they are already at a stage of growth that normally takes place only within the biliary tract some time after the metacercariae have reached that goal and begun to grow into the mature animal.

There is a rare piece of confirmatory evidence that the parasites in some cases are immature liver flukes: visceral fascioliasis, in the form of infestation of the trachea and bronchi, with the risk of secondary bacterial pneumonia and abscess formation, has followed halzoun.* I have known one such patient and his metazoan pests, as he called them, since the latter were found in an excised lung abscess and gave a fresh point to the history of the former's culinary experiences as a social anthropologist on field work in the Middle East.

Fascioliasis?

There is information on the liver fluke and the disease it ordinarily causes in the chapter before this one.

Linguatuliasis?

There will be information on the 'tongue worm' and its tropical relatives in the chapter on spiders in the prostate gland in *Exotica* (Chapter 48). Briefly, *Linguatula serrata,* the 'tongue worm', is an obligate endoparasite, the adults dwelling in the nasal passages of carnivores, particularly dogs, and the nymphs, or pentastome larvae, in the tissues of herbivores. The encysted first stage larvae are occasionally found in man, rarely causing harm. The third stage larvae are those concerned in halzoun.

Reference

(1)   Schacher, J. F., Saab, S., Germanos, R. & Boustany, N. (1969) The aetiology of halzoun in Lebanon: recovery of *Linguatula serrata* nymphs from two patients. *Transactions of the Royal Society of Tropical Medicine and Hygiene, 63* (November), 854–8.

* Bronchopulmonary fascioliasis occurring in such circumstances, or in any circumstances, has nothing, of course, to do with the usual form of pulmonary distomatosis, which is caused by *Paragonimus westermani* and endemic in many parts of eastern Asia.

19 The Hives at QCH

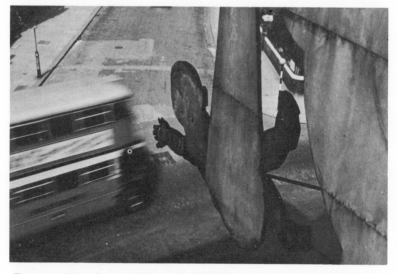

Fig. 19.1 'Stop the world—*I* want to get on!'
An outlook, and a viewpoint, at Queen Charlotte's Hospital on the Marylebone Road, in August, 1938. (*Photograph by W. St C. Symmers*)

It was customary in the old Queen Charlotte's Hospital in St Marylebone for all the medical students in residence to be summoned to see any especially unusual case, whether they were on call to attend the next deliveries or not. One morning the bell sounded at three, when most of us had been on the go for two nights and a day of uninterrupted progress toward the General Medical Council's required number of personally conducted confinements. The cause for this call had been the admission of a young Cockney primigravida whose time, gestationally speaking, had come. When she arrived in the labour ward she was found to have a delicate eruption of rose-coloured spots. This observation was compounded with fever, a slow pulse and her meridional husband's occupation as an itinerant *gelatiere*—the product was a tentative diagnosis of typhoid.

There was nothing else remarkable about the patient's condition. We had been called because the RMO, mindful of our general education in Medicine, felt we might not have the chance to see typhoid again in our hygienic age (it was the late 1930s). To a student from Ireland, at that time, a case of typhoid offered little novelty, even in pregnancy: for, though the disease was something of a rarity there too, we saw enough of it to have clerked cases with some regularity in the general wards of the teaching hospitals in Belfast as well as in the Purdysburn Fever Hospital. I slipped back to my room and slept again while the others sleepily considered rose spots, fetal heart sounds, incubation periods and whether to call at the Inoculation Department for a TAB when we gate-crashed St Mary's swimming bath later in the day.

As it happened, the patient had hives, not typhoid, and her recovery was quick, uncomplicated and accompanied by the arrival of a son.

Footnote. I imagine that some of that group of midwifery students must later have had wry occasion to remember the RMO's optimistic belief in the imminent eradication of typhoid. But it was the era of Prontosil, Bayer's pioneer sulphonamide (already changing from red to white),* and of the Colebrooks' contributions at Queen Charlotte's to the 'chemical cure' of puerperal sepsis due to Lancefield group A β-haemolytic streptococci. Few could have foreseen the ex-

---

* Prontosil Rubrum, the first marketed sulphonamide, soon gave place to the simpler, safer and more effective Prontosil Album (sulphanilamide).

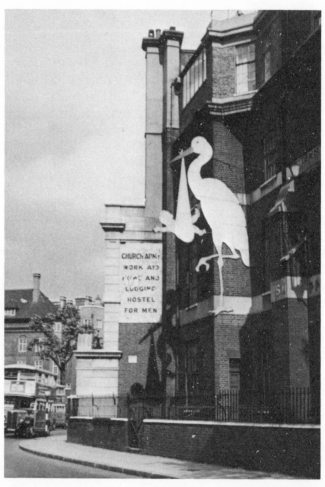

Fig. 19.2.   QCH, Marylebone Road—August, 1938. After the hospital moved wholly to its Goldhawk Road site in Hammersmith, the old buildings eventually became the headquarters of St Dunstan's, for men and women blinded on war service: this is its present role . . .   (*Photograph by W. St C. Symmers*)

tent to which infections were quite soon to come under the
control of chemotherapy, and the antibiotics were still undiscovered. That RMO (who was not himself a Mary's man)
was right, in principle, when he told us that one day some one
in what he referred to as 'that place along the road', on Praed
Street, would find a Prontosil for typhoid . . . Maybe it has
been a far road from Prontosil to chloramphenicol and ampi-
cillin, but near its start were St Mary's and Fleming.

20 'Typhus is a Disease of Foreigners'★

Once, when it was one of my duties to examine candidates
for employment by the state and determine their fitness for
enlistment, I declared a woman to be medically fit who turned
out to be a typhoid carrier. She had recently arrived from
another European country. She had no symptoms of any
kind. When I took her history she told me she had had typhus
two years earlier. This seemed reasonable, for at that time she
had been in a war-riven land where louse-borne rickettsial
typhus fever had been a problem.

It did not occur to me that in fact she meant typhoid fever,
enteric fever, caused by *Salmonella typhi*. But in her country,
as in many others in Europe, what in English is referred to as
typhoid fever (the 'typhoid'—typhus-like—fever) is known
as typhus abdominalis (typhus, for short), while what we call
typhus is typhus exanthematicus (typhus exanthematicus, for

★ Thus a British medical student of the seventies (the 1970s), in an answer to a question in the
Final MB examination paper.
     There were five questions on the paper, for which three hours were allowed. One of the
five was: 'Write a short note (not more than 100 words) on each of the following . . .?'
One of the five topics in this 'short-note' question was *Typhus Fever*. The candidate
whose answer is reproduced *verbatim* in the title of this chapter did better in the rest of the
paper, and passed.

short—sometimes just typhus). There was no excuse for the mistake: these Latin terms for the two diseases are in the books —they are even in my lecture notes from student days.

By public good fortune, the new recruit was not the source of any cases of the infection (or, if she was, they were never recognized). A week after my examination, already in her new job, she developed acute appendicitis. As there was a little looseness of the stools while she was in hospital after the appendicectomy, cultures were made and *Salmonella typhi* was grown. It was then realized that it was typhoid that she had had two years before.

Her carrier state appeared to be exclusively alimentary. It eventually cleared up when her gall bladder was removed (this was well before the days of antityphoid antibiotics). The acute appendicitis was considered to have been coincidental.

Rocket. The woman's first name, anglicized, was Mary. At the enquiry into the circumstances that had allowed a typhoid carrier to be passed fit for service, the non-medical but medically advised president maintained that any doctor familiar with the history of the best known of all typhoid carriers, 'Typhoid Mary', should have been alerted to the possibility of this state by the fact that the recruit bore the same name, Mary. When the reprimand was at last promulgated, this view was confirmed as contributory evidence of neglectful performance of medical duties.

Mary III

Another woman translated her name to Mary when she came to join her husband on his demobilization in Britain in 1946. Their children being old enough not to need her full attention, she resumed the work that she had been trained for and became a catering officer. She had held this job successfully for some years when an attack of biliary colic led to her admission to the hospital for treatment. While she was in the ward, her husband went sick with what turned out to be typhoid fever. His illness was a mild one, probably because he had been immunized with TAB on many occasions during military service in the 1939–45 war. The source of his infection was a puzzle: he had not been abroad since the war, and there were no other recognized cases of typhoid in the country at the time of his attack.

When his wife, herself still in the hospital as a patient, heard what was wrong with him, she disclosed that, while still in her own country, she had been found to be a persistent carrier of typhoid, the sequel of an attack of the disease during a war-time epidemic. Since that time she had relied on her own fastidious personal hygiene to prevent passing the infection to others. It grieved her greatly that in the end she had failed—there could be little doubt that she was the source of her husband's illness. This history known, her stools were cultured: *Salmonella typhi* was grown. The treatment of her biliary symptoms included cholecystectomy because of gall stones: the typhoid bacillus was isolated from the stones also. After the operation, repeated attempts to grow the organism again from faecal and other specimens were consistently unsuccessful.

There were no further cases. This Mary seems no longer to be a typhoid Mary. Nevertheless, she is the first to agree that she will not return to catering work.

21 Dangerous Drug

One of a familiar breed, the peripatetic university examiner,* having finished his main job, was invited by an organization for cultural relations to make a short lecture tour in the region. The tour included a visit to the beautiful modern hospital that, with architectural justification, was a show-piece of one of the fascinating cities on his itinerary. Unfortunately, through shortage of funds, it had never been possible to employ the skilled staff necessary to make use of all the facilities that the buildings were so well provided with: whole departments remained unopened, decaying from disuse and lack of maintenance.

Parts of the hospital were very old, the shabby remnants of an honourable endeavour by a former government to meet its responsibilities. Among the oldest buildings was the isolation wing. The examiner, blind-eyed to his guide's protesting gesture, walked over to the wing, his attention caught by the photographic possibilities of the style and material. On the screen-door of one of the isolation wards was a red ribbon, tied to form a Latin cross, perhaps a surviving recollection of an age-old talisman that should both warn and protect in the presence of pestilence. Peering through the wire mesh, the examiner saw a solitary nurse, sitting by the cot of a deathly still child whose brow she was sponging. Four other children

---

* Further misadventures of the extern examiner—this one or some of his fellows?—are scattered through these volumes, among others particularly in Chapters 7 and 8 of the third book, *Memorata*. There is one on page 153 of this volume.

72

lay in other cots, two motionless, two plucking feebly with their fingers, at nothing.

The examiner asked his companion what the children were ill with. 'Typhoid', was the answer, 'They're dying of typhoid'. The examiner was puzzled. 'Is it a resistant strain?', he asked, uncertain whether the typhoid bacillus in fact might show antibiotic resistance* but unable to think how else the evident lack of response to treatment could be explained. 'Resistant to what?', asked the other in reply, with a Gallic gesture of resignation, 'There's nothing specific we can use, after all.' 'I meant chloramphenicol', said the examiner (it was before the 'new' penicillins). 'Oh', said the local man, 'But we don't use chloramphenicol . . . It's far too toxic to the bone marrow.'

It appeared that the hospital had a list of Standing Regulations and Instructions (a relic of former times, perhaps). One of the contemporary Additions and Emendations was that the use of chloramphenicol was absolutely forbidden because of the risk of fatal depression of the bone marrow. The hospital's pharmacy was not allowed to keep a stock of the drug. The examiner was able to get a good supply from one of the foreign embassies in the town (not his own—the duty officer was appalled by the idea of such interference in the affairs of a friendly government and would not disclose the whereabouts of the 'embassy' doctor). It was too late for two of the children.

The head of the hospital was displeased that a visitor had meddled in the care of patients. He reported the matter to various authorities whom he presumably thought to have disciplinary powers: but the extern examiner has not been made to regard what he did as regrettable, though it is true that he no longer contributes officially to cultural relations between his country and others.

* It may.

22 Wonder Drug

A young man was admitted to hospital for surgical treatment of an uncomplicated inguinal hernia. He mentioned to the house surgeon that he had pain while urinating. The house-man was able to express a droplet of pus from the patient's urinary meatus and made a film of it which was sent to the laboratory for examination. The laboratory report was that gonococci were present. A single intramuscular injection of 300 000 units of procaine penicillin was prescribed (at that time still ordinarily a curative dose in cases of acute gonorrhoea in that country).

The injection was given into the left buttock by a staff nurse. She had just used the same syringe to give an intra-muscular injection of penicillin to another newly admitted patient, a diabetic with acute appendicitis and chronic furunculosis. The diabetic's boils had been no more than a recurring nuisance to him. His general practitioner's attempts to control them with penicillin and tetracyclines had been un-successful: laboratory tests had shown the responsible staphy-lococcus to be resistant to these drugs. Unfortunately, the house surgeon had not been told by the GP about these findings: on general principles, therefore, he ordered a course of penicillin to minimize the chances of staphylococcal sepsis complicating the imminent appendicectomy.

Although the nurse changed needles between the injections she did not use a fresh syringe, for she believed penicillin solution itself to be 'strong' enough to disinfect such apparatus. She had used a new needle, partly because the first one had

74

seemed rather blunt, partly because she knew there was a chance of passing hepatitis virus from patient to patient if the needle was not changed between injections . . . In accordance with her training, to ensure that the needle was not in a blood vessel she had pulled on the plunger of the syringe before making each injection.

The patient with the hernia developed an acute abscess in the left buttock. Its presence was recognized on the day after the herniorrhaphy, which was performed two days after his admission to the hospital. Cultures of the pus grew *Staphylococcus aureus* of the same phage type as that responsible for the diabetic patient's boils: it was resistant to penicillin, streptomycin, tetracycline, chloramphenicol and erythromycin, which at that time effectively exhausted the range of antibiotics immediately available. He died of fulminating staphylococcal septicaemia on the eighth day after the injection.

The diabetic patient's convalescence from his appendicectomy was straightforward. No other cases of sepsis due to his staphylococcus were recognized in the hospital.

Comment

The circumstantial evidence that the infection was introduced when the injection of penicillin was given can scarcely be set aside. It is horrifying to have to admit that trained staff may not understand the practical application of the elementary principles of asepsis. But our lives in hospital are as much in the hands of the innocently ignorant as at the mercy of the culpably irresponsible.

Reference

(1)   Symmers, W. St C. (1965) Infections as complications of drug therapy—with summaries of seventeen cases of viral, bacterial, fungal and protozoal

infection. In *Drug-Induced Diseases—Second Symposium Organized by the Boerhaave Courses for Post-Graduate Medical Education—State University of Leyden, October 1954*, edited by L. Meyler and H. M. Peck, pages 108–51. Amsterdam, New York, London, Milan, Tokyo and Buenos Aires: Excerpta Medica Foundation.

23 An Opportunistic Infection: A Fatal Case of Athlete's Foot[1]

An opportunist is a person who, meeting an unusual or unexpected environmental circumstance, turns the meeting to his advantage.

An opportunistic infection is caused by a micro-organism that, meeting an unusual environmental circumstance, is able by reason of this circumstance to establish itself in progressive parasitism in the body of a host that otherwise would have been immune from invasion to such depth and extent by that organism.

The concept of 'opportunistic infections' seems to date from 1954, when Professor Heinz Seeliger, then in Bonn, wrote of the fungi that cause pulmonary mycoses[2]:

> *Bei der Mehrzahl der angeschuldigten Pilze handelt es sich um ausgesprochene* Opportunisten, *die erst nach einer Störung des biologischen Gleichgewichts ihre schädlichen Wirkungen entfalten.* (The majority of the fungi blamed [for these infections] are frank *opportunists* that disclose their harmful effects only after a disturbance of the biological equilibrium.*)

* Dr John P. Utz, of Richmond, Virginia, has pointed out that a concept that ascribes to micro-organisms the volitional characteristic of opportunism is teleological.[3] This is

The case that follows illustrates the 'disturbance of biological equilibrium' between host and micro-organism that characteristically leads to progressive, fatal infection by an organism that ordinarily causes no more than local, even trivial, disease.

Case[1]

A man of 63 developed chronic lymphatic leukaemia. He was treated with tretamine, which controlled the disease reasonably well.

He had long had 'athlete's foot', caused by *Trichophyton rubrum*. The fungus was also responsible for a mild, chronic tinea elsewhere on his limbs and trunk. Apart from the occasional use of an antifungal dusting powder he had never bothered with treatment for the infection.

He had quite severe varicose veins in both legs.

Six months after starting treatment for leukaemia the patient was lecturing to a learned society when he slipped off the edge of the low platform, sustaining a Pott's fracture of one ankle. The bone was set and a plaster of Paris cast applied. The plaster was too tight, causing a pressure ulcer to develop over the medial malleolus. The ulcer did not heal, probably because of the poor circulation associated with the varicose veins: instead, it spread to the shin and became transformed into a chronic varicose ulcer. The patient refused to have treatment for either the varicosities or the ulcer, other than to keep the latter covered with a dry dressing under a simple bandage.

Ten months after the fracture he met a surgeon socially whom he had not previously known. He told the surgeon

---

valid criticism: how much more valid when an abstraction—infection—is designated 'opportunistic'. Still, 'opportunistic infection' remains a term without any succinct alternative: and it has become accepted as indicating the infections—increasingly important and frequent and various as they are—that result from a growing range of influences capable of eroding the body's defences.

about the ulcer. Incredibly, the latter, without thought that the patient was under the care of other doctors, and without examining him, suggested that he take hydrocortisone by mouth, in view of his refusal to consider any other form of treatment. The patient had not mentioned that he was under treatment for leukaemia.

About a month after starting on hydrocortisone he noticed that part of the ulcer was becoming angrier. He drew this to the attention of the physician who was dealing with the leukaemia, but he did not tell him about the surgeon's prescription for hydrocortisone. The physician arranged for a biopsy. The sections showed mycelium in the necrotic floor of the ulcer (Fig. 23.1). *Trichophyton rubrum* was grown from the ulcer.

Two weeks or so after the biopsy the inguinal lymph nodes of that side became swollen and painful. Biopsy showed

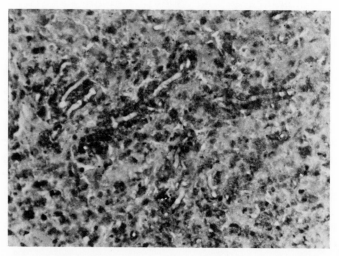

Fig. 23.1.   The floor of the varicose ulcer is necrotic tissue. Mycelium is seen tracking through the field, covered by a rather narrow deposit of partly haematoxyphile, partly eosinophile matter that may be similar in significance to the more hyaline material of the candida asteroid illustrated in Fig. 2.2 (page 8).[4]

Haematoxylin–eosin   × 360

lymphosarcomatous replacement of the normal structure of the nodes, with extensive necrosis. In addition, there were hyphae in the necrotic tissue and passing through the walls of thrombosed blood vessels, particularly in the capsule of the nodes (Fig. 23.2). Cultures from one of the nodes gave a pure growth of *Trichophyton rubrum*.

The patient's condition deteriorated rapidly. He died in coma three weeks after the lymph node biopsy. As well as

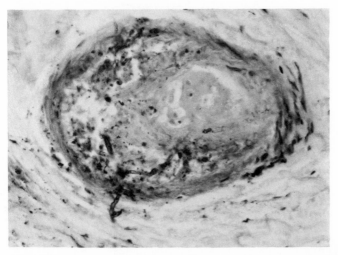

Fig. 23.2.   This small vein, in tissue adjoining one of the excised inguinal lymph nodes, is obliterated by fresh thrombus. There are hyphae of the fungus in the thrombus and penetrating the wall of the vessel. While it would not be possible to identify the genus of the fungus from its appearances in the cutaneous ulcer (Fig. 23.1) and in this specimen, the isolation of *Trichophyton rubrum* from both sites makes this identification reasonably likely, particularly as the same organism was grown in pure culture from lesions in many of the viscera *post mortem* (see Fig. 23.3). It can be assumed that the fungus was carried in lymph to the groin, where—perhaps because of the obstruction to the flow through the nodes caused by the necrotic lymphosarcoma—it established infection and spread through the tissues to reach and invade veins, so setting up the fatal trichophyton septicaemia.

Reproduced by permission of the Editor of the *American Journal of Clinical Pathology* (the illustration was originally published in the article cited as Reference 1 on page 82).

Periodic-acid/Schiff: haemalum   × 360

chronic leukaemia and lymphosarcomatosis, the PM showed many necrotic foci in various organs, including the brain (Fig. 23.3). Pure cultures of *Trichophyton rubrum* were obtained from these foci.

Comment

This is a classic example of an 'opportunistic' infection. The infections that may be so called are caused by organisms that

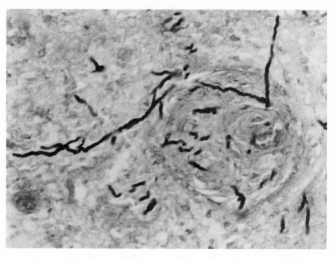

Fig. 23.3.   Fungal hyphae radiating into brain tissue from a small thrombosed and infected blood vessel. Again, the identification of the organism as the trichophyton is presumptive (see caption of Fig. 23.2). In contrast to Fig. 23.1, there is no precipitate round the hyphae in this illustration or in Fig. 23.2.

*Hexamine–silver**   × 300

* Why import methenamine when hexamine is a local product? And why, in places where the usual name for hexamethylenetetramine is hexamine, use methenamine (the word) when referring to the use of methenamine (the substance) in connexion with this most valuable means of demonstrating fungi in histological sections ('Grocott's stain for fungi'—the 'methenamine silver nitrate method' or, as it is the same thing chemically, the 'hexamine-silver method')?

Methenamine is the official name in the United States National Formulary for the urinary antiseptic that the British Pharmaceutical Codex officially calls hexamine. Imported methenamine, used by some British labs, costs a hundred times as much as hexamine supplied by British purveyors of fine laboratory chemicals: both are the same hexamethylenetetramine.

ordinarily have limited or no pathogenic capacity, yet can cause serious, progressive disease as a result of changes in the body's resistance (see below).[5] *Trichophyton rubrum* is one of the common, important dermatophytes, the fungi that cause superficial mycoses, confined to the epidermis, hair and nails. Very occasionally, like other species of trichophyton, it causes suppurative cutaneous folliculitis and perifolliculitis, but extension of infection beyond the skin is so rare that the case described in this chapter is one of only two or three published instances of proven septicaemic trichophytosis. One of the notable implications of such cases is that the trichophyta—ordinarily keratinophile organisms—can adapt themselves to thrive in the deeper tissues of the body, where keratin is not available.

The organisms that cause opportunistic infections include bacteria, fungi, viruses and protozoa.* Such infections are predisposed to both by diseases that lower resistance through interfering with the cellular or humoral defences and by the comparable side effects of therapeutic measures. Precisely how this predisposition is mediated is still largely unknown.

The predisposing diseases include systemic diseases of the lymphoreticular system (particularly Hodgkin's disease), leukaemia, severe anaemia, granulocytopenia, hypogamma-globulinaemia, malnutrition, cachexia, severe metabolic disorders and chronic renal and hepatic insufficiencies. The therapeutic agents that have a comparable effect include radiotherapy, cytotoxic drugs, immunosuppressants, cor-ticosteroids and, in certain circumstances, broad-spectrum

---

* In one case,[6] to be described in the third volume of this series, *Memorata* (Chapter 26), the patient died with four generalized haematogenous fungal infections (aspergillosis, candidosis, phycomycosis and cryptococcosis), generalized cytomegalovirus infection and a widespread protozoal pneumonia (*Pneumocystis carinii* infection) as well as a non-opportunistic staphylococcal pneumonia and pyaemia. The predisposing conditions were longstanding Hodgkin's disease (complicated by autoimmune haemolytic anaemia and terminal acute leukaemia) and the side effects of treatment with X-rays, cytotoxic drugs and corticosteroids.

antibiotics. Prolonged or repeated canulation of the vasculature, haemodialysis and extracorporeal circulation—also important in this context—act mainly as potential sources of infection.

Particular Case. In the case described here there was the characteristic combination of prepared soil and abundant seed. Tissue resistance to invasion by the fungus was lowered through the combined effects of leukaemia, cytotoxic therapy and hydrocortisone. Development of the ulcer of the shin presented the trichophyton, already long established on the skin, with access to the now vulnerable deeper tissues.

References

(1)   Symmers, W. St C. (1966) Deep-seated fungal infections currently seen in the histopathologic service of a medical school laboratory in Britain. *American Journal of Clinical Pathology, 46* (November), 514–37.
(2)   Seeliger, H. (1954) Die Lungenmykosen und ihre Immunbiologie. *Medizinische Monatsschrift, 8* (October), 692–8.
(3)   Utz, J. P. (1962) The spectrum of opportunistic fungus infections. *Laboratory Investigation, 11* (November), 1018–25.
(4)   Symmers, W. St C. (1972) Histopathology of phycomycoses. *Annales de la Société Belge de Médecine Tropicale, 52,* 365–88.
(5)   Symmers, W. St C. (1965) The concept of 'opportunistic infections'. *Proceedings of the Royal Society of Medicine, 58* (May), 341–6.
(6)   Symmers, W. St C. (1965) Infections as complications of drug therapy—with summaries of seventeen cases of viral, bacterial, fungal and protozoal infection. In *Drug-Induced Diseases—Second Symposium Organized by the Boerhaave Courses for Post-Graduate Medical Education—State University of Leyden, October 1954,* edited by L. Meyler and H. M. Peck, pages 108–51. Amsterdam, New York, London, Milan, Tokyo and Buenos Aires: Excerpta Medica Foundation.

24 A Case of Toxoplasmosis . . .

(not Hodgkin's Disease)

A medical student at the start of his first hospital year went to
a clinic on Hodgkin's disease. Next day, fearing that this was
the explanation of the firm, enlarged lymph nodes that he
had been aware of for some weeks in both sides of his neck,
he called on the doctor in charge of the student health service.
Biopsy of a node followed: the report was early Hodgkin's
disease and treatment with X-rays was begun.

The student did not feel ill, but he was greatly disturbed by
the diagnosis, the more so as he had just become engaged to be
married. His parents had recently moved to another city: the
university there agreed, on compassionate grounds, to accept
him as a clinical student. He completed the initial course of
X-rays and then moved to his new school, where, a few days
later, he was seen by the head of the radiotherapy department.
The latter, in accordance with a wise custom of reviewing the
histological specimens of all patients referred from other
hospitals for treatment, arranged for sections of the student's
node to be obtained from the centre where the diagnosis of
Hodgkin's disease had been made.

The pathologist who reviewed the sections considered the
appearances typical of toxoplasmosis. The results of the complement fixation and dye tests were confirmatory, showing
titres of 1 : 16 and 1 : 1024 respectively. There was no histological evidence of Hodgkin's disease, this diagnosis having

been based on misinterpretation of the classic picture of toxo-plasmic lymphadenitis (Figs 24.1 and 24.2).

It was some time before the patient accepted that he had been suffering from merely a benign, self-limiting, infective lymphadenopathy.

The radiotherapy, which had been confined to the

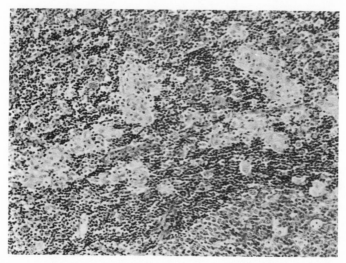

Fig. 24.1. Toxoplasmic lymphadenitis varies considerably in its range of histological pictures. One consequence is that the condition tends to be overlooked when it happens not to have given rise to changes that immediately bring its classic microscopical picture to mind. But even the latter may be misinterpreted, particularly as it has some similarity to the changes in some early cases of sarcoid-osis and of Hodgkin's disease. The field in this illustration is representative of what was present throughout the student's lymph node: it shows the clustered pale macrophages forming the characteristically small and 'geographically' outlined foci that must always suggest the possibility of this infection and the need therefore to arrange for the appropriate serological investigations. Some-times, of course, it is impossible to find confirmatory evidence of toxoplasmosis: whatever disease the patient has may subside without its cause being identified, or, occasionally, its progress eventually indicates another diagnosis. As such 'other diagnosis' may prove to be Hodgkin's disease, it is not surprising that, conversely, this interpretation is sometimes mistakenly put forward, as in the student's case, when events are to show toxoplasmosis to be responsible. See Fig. 24.2 also.

Haematoxylin–eosin × 120

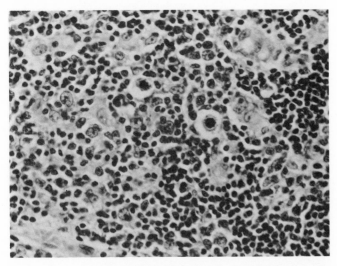

Fig. 24.2. This sort of field, from the vicinity of characteristic lesions of
toxoplasmosis in the node, seems to have been responsible for the mistaken
original diagnosis of Hodgkin's disease. As well as a scattering of single reticulum
cells and of small clusters of epithelioid macrophages, there are here two cells in
mitosis, both appearing as heavily stained compact nuclei with cytoplasm that
has shrunk to leave a rather large space between the cell and the surroundings.
It is when such fields suggest the possibility of a malignant condition that the
pathologist may find it increasingly difficult to escape from making a possibility
into a diagnosis.

Haematoxylin–eosin   × 300

posterior triangles of his neck, had no recognized effect,
disadvantageous (see page 92) or otherwise, on the course of
the infection.

Comment

Like language, manners and customs, diseases change with
the times. This present-day student was eventually interested
to learn something of the experiences he might have had
under similar circumstances in the days of his teachers'
generation. In the 1930s, in Ireland at least, we discovered

(mostly through the worries of our afflicted fellows) that what medical students supposed to be Hodgkin's disease in themselves was likely to be either tuberculous lymphadenitis, or the lymphadenitis of what we knew as 'abortus fever' (infection by *Brucella abortus*), or glandular fever (infectious mononucleosis). Sometimes, of course, it was just a non-specific lymphadenitis associated with some focus of chronic inflammation about the mouth or throat.

Now, thirty years and more on, the students whom we teach seem as prone as we were to misinterpret any personal lymphadenopathy of more than a few days' duration as Hodgkin's disease. Tuberculosis is no longer a cause of their delusion, so far has milk-borne tuberculosis been eliminated in our community (it is over twenty years since I saw a student, raised in these islands, whose 'Hodgkin's disease' turned out to be Tb nodes). Non-specific chronic lymphadenitis, infectious mononucleosis (glandular fever) and, less frequently, brucellosis still bring students this anxiety, but between them they account for about half of the cases only: most of the rest have toxoplasmic lymphadenitis, an entity that was unrecognized until the 1950s.* It is hard to believe that we overlooked toxoplasmosis as a cause of lymphadenopathy for so long. Perhaps this protozoal infection is indeed becoming commoner, [1,2] but the histological picture characteristic of toxoplasmic lymphadenitis has certainly been familiar for a

---

* For some years during the 1950s, in Britain, the necrotizing lymphadenitis of cat-scratch fever was less rare than before then and since. It, too, accounted for some of the worry by students and young doctors, not to mention nurses, on the score of its clinical misinterpretation as Hodgkin's disease. Also, until pathologists became familiar with its occurrence, the histological picture of the 'stellate abscesses' led to a number of unfortunate biopsy reports of 'lymphogranuloma inguinale of the neck' (nomenclature surely as insensitive as the diagnosticians who adopted it).

Histological confusion between cat-scratch disease and lymphogranuloma inguinale is avoidable when one knows which disease the patient has. The clinical history helps, usually, and the intradermal antigen tests give the histologist useful support. The two diseases are generally believed to be caused by similar organisms of the chlamydial group.

A student, originally warned that she probably had Hodgkin's disease and then told that she had venereal infection of the cervical lymph nodes, took her life. It was cat-scratch disease that she had.

long time, if under other names;* our oversight has been the failure to recognize the role of the infective agent, though it has been known as a parasite of animals since 1908 and of man since 1923. Serological evidence shows that sub-clinical infection by the toxoplasma is extraordinarily wide-spread in man, whose source of disease still remains uncertain; congenital infection, usually without symptoms in the mother, is familiar in various grave forms, whereas acquired infection in the older child and adult is ordinarily symptomless and in only a small minority of cases presents with lymph-adenitis. Possibly animals, particularly domestic ones, are an important reservoir.

Protozoal Lymphadenitis. Many types of protozoa may occasionally infect lymph nodes, the resulting histological changes being specific only in so far as the organisms them-selves are recognizable in the tissues. It is particularly in-teresting that *Toxoplasma gondii* and *Leishmania*, both of them intracellular parasites with a predilection for the cells of the reticuloendothelial system, should cause the same striking pattern of small, discrete histiocytic aggregates in infected lymph nodes (and in other lymphoid tissues, such as the ton-sils): the only distinguishing feature is the demonstrable presence of the leishmanias in the histiocytes (see *Exotica,* Figs 13.3 and 13.4).

It is almost unknown for toxoplasmas to be demonstrated in conventional histological preparations of infected lymph nodes, even when they are readily isolatable from the nodes by the mouse inoculation procedure: the rarity of an observation such as that illustrated in Fig. 24.3 contrasts with the com-parative ease of demonstrating the organisms in visceral lesions of fatal cases of toxoplasmosis in infancy (and in adults whose

---

* Lymphohistiocytic medullary reticulosis of Robb-Smith, for instance, and the Piringer–Kuchinka lymphadenopathy—but not all the cases to which such terms may have been applicable have been instances of toxoplasmosis.

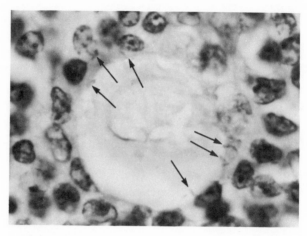

Fig. 24.3   The arrows point to single crescentic toxoplasmas at the periphery of what seems to be a large and disintegrating macrophage or reticulum cell. Several more toxoplasmas were seen at the same site when the section was examined at other planes of focus: none was found elsewhere in the node. It is very rare indeed for the organisms to be demonstrable in histological preparations of infected lymph nodes in cases of acquired toxoplasmic lymphadenitis, even though they may be readily isolated by inoculating material from the same specimens into the peritoneal cavity of mice. Compare this situation with that illustrated in Figs 24.4 and 24.5. See Figs 25.1 and 25.2 also (pages 93 and 94).
Haematoxylin–eosin   × 1300

resistance has been undermined—Figs 24.4 and 24.5). The explanation of this peculiar difference between the lesions of acquired toxoplasmic lymphadenitis, a usually benign condition, and those of fatal cerebral or generalized toxoplasmosis is unknown: it may prove to be an important step toward understanding the pathogenesis of the infection under different conditions of resistance and immunity.

Lymphadenopathy in Students

It is necessary to return, briefly, to the general topic. Once, perhaps over-aware that benign conditions cause students to fear that they have Hodgkin's disease, I reassured a young

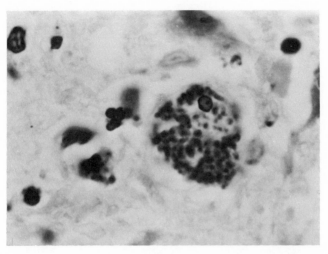

Fig. 24.4.   In cases of encephalitis due to infection with the toxoplasma, whether congenital or acquired, it is usually easy to find the parasites in the lesions. They may be numerous or scanty; cysts such as are illustrated here may be absent or conspicuous, and may indicate a certain chronicity of the infection. The toxoplasma is essentially an intracellular parasite, but is commonly seen free in the tissues while passing from cell to cell during the proliferative phase of infection or after release from the cysts and in search of host cells in which to resume the cycle. The cyst itself develops within a host cell: when the latter dies the parasitic structure lies free. The merozoites within the cyst are smaller and more rounded than the trophozoites of the proliferative phase (compare this figure and Fig. 24.5 with Figs 25.1 and 25.2 on pages 93 and 94). In the cyst shown in this picture the relatively large round structure may be the degenerate nucleus of the host cell, probably microglial in nature. Two neutrophils in the field contain individual toxoplasmas.

The patient whose infection was the source of this preparation was an adult under immunosuppressant treatment on account of a renal transplant. He died of rapidly progressive encephalitis. Whether this was reactivation of a dormant infection or followed exposure to exogenous infection is uncertain, but in either event it would be regarded as 'opportunistic' (see page 76).

Haematoxylin–eosin   × 1050

colleague too confidently before his biopsy operation. He had Hodgkin's disease, as well as the fear of it.

Later, I had to tell another student that her biopsied cervical node contained secondary deposits from an as yet undiscovered melanoma. She, too, had been afraid that the enlargement of the nodes meant that she had Hodgkin's disease,

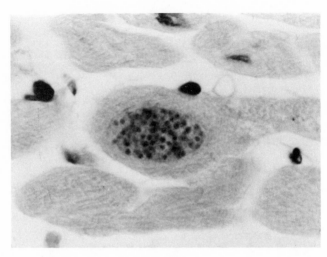

Fig. 24.5 A retired parasitologist died in an accident. The photograph shows an intact parasitic cyst in a myocardial fibre, one of scanty identical cysts in sections of the only block of tissue available for examination, part of the wall of the left ventricle. Specific fluorescent-antibody studies confirmed that the organism is *Toxoplasma gondii* and not one of the other parasites that may infect muscle and be mistaken for toxoplasma—for instance, *Trypanosoma cruzi* (the cause of American trypanosomiasis—Chagas's disease) and species of *Nosema* (*Encephalitozoon*), *Sarcocystis* and the like.

Haematoxylin–eosin × 1500

and a kindly doctor had told her that the biopsy would show that she had no need to worry. The primary was a minute tumour in the scalp.

*　　*　　*

An Afterthought: Contemporary Pathology, and a Contemporary Courtesy. I was asked to another teaching hospital to see a patient who was thought to have toxoplasmic lymphadenitis. It was 1965, or thereabouts. When I got to the ward, the staff nurse in charge—attractive, friendly and efficient—was filing papers in the duty room. She took me down the ward to meet the patient. As we went behind the screens round the bed, I asked the nurse if she would mind putting her cigarette out while we were with the patient—'Gosh, no', she replied, 'Of course not, if it bothers you', and, with a smile, she stubbed it in the ashtray on the patient's locker before introducing us.

References

(1) Beattie, C. P. (1967) Toxoplasmosis. In *Recent Advances in Medical Micro-biology*, edited by A. P. Waterson, chapter 9, pages 318–51. London: Churchill.
(2) Beverley, J. K. A. (1960) The laboratory diagnosis of toxoplasmosis. In *Recent Advances in Clinical Pathology*, Series 3, edited by S. C. Dyke, Mary Barber, E. N. Allott, Rosemary Biggs and A. H. T. Robb-Smith, chapter 4, pages 38–57. London: Churchill.

25 ... and a Case of Toxoplasmosis ...

(and Hodgkin's Disease)[1,2]

Protozoa are among the rarer causes of 'opportunistic' infections (page 76). Least infrequent of such protozoa is *Pneumocystis carinii*, occasionally causing opportunistic pneumonia in adults, particularly when they have been treated for long periods with large doses of corticosteroids. The resulting infection is similar to the interstitial pneumocystis pneumonia with intra-alveolar parasitosis that is the familiar manifestation of pneumocystis infection in infancy, when the predisposing circumstance is prematurity or other cause of failure to thrive. Interestingly, pneumocystis pneumonia in babies (and, exceptionally, in adults[3]) is often accompanied by generalized cytomegalovirus infection—a peculiar symbiosis of protozoon and virus. Next to the pneumocystis in frequency among opportunistic protozoa are the amoebae, particularly *Entamoeba coli*.

In the case described in this chapter, the protozoon was *Toxoplasma gondii*. As in the case of the medical student (page 83), the initial evidence of the infection was the usual toxoplasmic cervical lymphadenitis: but, instead of subsiding, the disease was progressive, ending fatally with the occurrence —unprecedented in man—of peritonitis with massive effusion. The patient had Hodgkin's disease and was under treatment with X-rays, nitrogen mustard and hydrocortisone. It can scarcely be denied that the uncharacteristic course and outcome of the infection were attributable to these resistance-lowering factors.

History

The patient was forty-six when he was found to have Hodgkin's disease. His course of treatment with X-rays and mustine spread over the following five years, until his death from toxoplasmosis.

Four years after recognition of his Hodgkin's disease he developed thrombocytopenic purpura. Antiplatelet antibodies were found. Treatment with fifty milligrams of hydrocortisone daily by mouth generally kept the platelet count well above the purpura level, but occasional outbreaks of petechial bleeding required the dose to be raised temporarily. Attempts to wean him off the steroid were unsuccessful, regularly resulting in severe thrombocytopenic episodes.

Five months after starting treatment with hydrocortisone he had a recurrence of enlargement of the lymph nodes in one side of the neck. Biopsy of one of these nodes showed no evidence of Hodgkin's disease but instead the picture ordinarily associated with acquired toxoplasmic lymphadenitis. The diagnosis of toxoplasmosis was confirmed by a rising titre in the dye and complement fixation tests. Reviewing the original biopsy specimens of almost five years before showed the picture of the fully developed classic form of Hodgkin's disease: there was no trace in the sections that toxoplasmosis had been present then (the contrary would have been unlikely, but knowledge of the duration of active toxoplasmosis in adults is still far from complete, and the negative finding is of note).

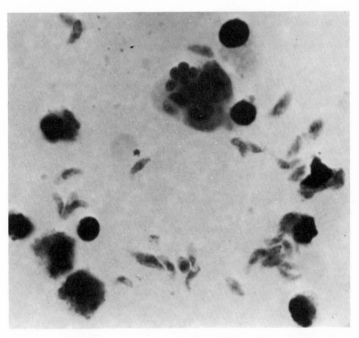

Fig. 25.1   This and Fig. 25.2 are photographs of a film of the patient's peritoneal exudate obtained by aspiration on the day before his death. The fluid was spread on the microscope slides as it came from the needle, without centrifugation. Many crescentic toxoplasmas are seen. There is also a freshly ruptured cyst (top, centre): it contains several distinctly rounded parasitic cells (merozoites). Compare with Figs 24.4 and 24.5 (pages 89 and 90).

Reproduced by permission of the Honorary Editors of the *Proceedings of the Royal Society of Medicine* (the illustration was originally published in the article cited as Reference 2 on page 95).

Haematoxylin–eosin   × 1300

A course of pyrimethamine was started, this antimalarial being known to have some effect on toxoplasmosis. The dose was twenty-five milligrams daily, by mouth. The drug had to be stopped because of the early appearance of severe thrombocytopenia and purpura, a recognized side effect that had been anticipated in view of the patient's existing tendency to drop his platelet count.

Four months after the diagnosis of toxoplasmosis, while still under treatment with X-rays, nitrogen mustard and

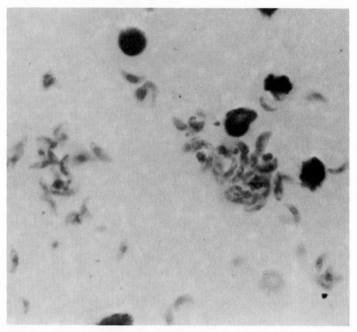

Fig. 25.2.   This field of the same preparation as Fig. 25.1 shows the crescentic trophozoites more clearly. The large size of the crescents in comparison with those illustrated at the same magnification in Fig. 24.3 (page 88) is due to the different methods of preparation of the two specimens: distortion by shrinkage is appreciably less in films of exudate than in paraffin sections of tissue processed by conventional histological means.

Haematoxylin–eosin   × 1300

hydrocortisone, the patient complained of abdominal discomfort. At first nothing was found to account for this, but within a few days progressive distension was apparent. After a week there was marked ascites and general abdominal tenderness. The patient went into a typhoid state of fever, delirium and collapse.

Examination of the peritoneal fluid (Figs 25.1 and 25.2) showed appearances identical with those in the exudate in laboratory animals after intraperitoneal inoculation of *Toxoplasma gondii* (the peritoneal inoculation test in mice is a standard procedure, occasionally necessary for proving the presence of the toxoplasma in material thought to be infected by it). Peritoneal toxoplasmosis in man has not been recorded in other cases.

The patient died a few days later. There was no PM.

References

(1) Symmers, W. St C. (1965) Infections as complications of drug therapy—with summaries of seventeen cases of viral, bacterial, fungal and protozoal infection. In *Drug-Induced Diseases—Second Symposium Organized by the Boerhaave Courses for Post-Graduate Medical Education—State University of Leyden, October 1954*, edited by L. Meyler and H. M. Peck, pages 108–51. Amsterdam, New York, London, Milan, Tokyo and Buenos Aires: Excerpta Medica Foundation.

(2) Symmers, W. St C. (1965) The concept of 'opportunistic infections'. *Proceedings of the Royal Society of Medicine, 58* (May), 341–6.

(3) Symmers, W. St C. (1960) Generalized cytomegalic inclusion-body disease associated with pneumocystis pneumonia in adults—a report of three cases, with Wegener's granulomatosis, thrombotic purpura, and Hodgkin's disease as predisposing conditions. *Journal of Clinical Pathology, 13* (January), 1–21.

26 ... Then One of Histoplasmosis ...[1]

This case of histoplasmosis is not remarkable so much because it is unusual as because the circumstance of its recognition so persuasively demonstrated the worthwhileness of reporting single cases of rare conditions (or of unusual manifestations of common ones). It was diagnosed because an editor had thought a case report worth publishing that three colleagues had thought worth writing,[2] and because a dentist* enjoys keeping up with the literature of a related profession, and regularly does so.

Histoplasmosis is both rare and common. It is rare in the experience of any doctor working in north-western Europe, indeed in any part of Europe, for the fungus that causes it, *Histoplasma capsulatum*, is native to only very limited regions of our continent. In contrast, in many parts of the world it is a common disease, as common even as tuberculosis has ever been. So, to some readers the account that follows will concern what they regard as a rare condition and to others it will describe merely a somewhat unusual manifestation of a common one: to appropriate a colleague's Hibernicism,† this common disease is quite rare.

Case

An Irishman, aged fifty-six, who had worked in India for thirty years, retired to Britain at the end of 1959. Early in the

---

* The dentist insists on his anonymity.
† Dr Sh-r-: "This common disease is quite rare".' *Charing Cross Hospital Gazette*, 1957 (October), 55, 236.

next year he went to his dentist because of an ulcer near the tip of his tongue, which he blamed on a habit of working it against a rough-edged filling in a molar tooth. He first noticed the ulcer about two years before leaving India: it healed then, spontaneously, and recurred in the same site; this sequence was repeated several times before he asked the dentist's advice.

The dentist described the ulcer as circular, about three millimetres across, and at the centre of a slightly raised area of induration about seven millimetres across. Its edge was well defined and rather redder than the normal mucosa nearby. Its floor was covered by greyish exudate that, when scraped away, left a hyperaemic ulcer.

The onset of his patient's chronic lingual ulcer while in India put the dentist in mind of a case that he had read about in a recent number of the *British Medical Journal*.[2] This was the case of an Englishman who had come home after thirty years in India and died of histoplasmosis that had caused massive destruction of the adrenals: his initial lesions had included an ulcer of the tongue (originally misdiagnosed histologically as a granular cell myoblastoma) and an anal granuloma (originally taken to be non-specific). The dentist did not really expect that his patient would prove to have histoplasmosis: but at least he was sure that the ulcer was no simple traumatic one.

The Specimen. The dentist excised the ulcer and the related zone of induration. He cut the specimen in two before sending it to the laboratory—one piece for culture and the other in formalin for histological examination. Unfortunately, the pathologist was not very familiar with fungi and in his apprehension exaggerated the difficulties and dangers associated with their isolation and identification. He wrote to the dentist that he lacked facilities for mycological work; disregarding that the dentist had told him that the whole lesion had been excised, he suggested taking another biopsy specimen and sending it to a mycologist—he added that he did not know of anyone working with fungi in England and therefore advised referring the problem to one of the most distinguished pioneers of medical mycology, a Frenchman (whom he did not know to have been dead for over twenty years). The dentist was too late to prevent the pathologist throwing away the specimen that had been intended for culture, but he was able to recover the formalin-fixed piece and send it to another laboratory where the sections were considered to be typical of histoplasmosis (Figs 26.1 and 26.2A).

Subsequent Course. At the time of diagnosis there were no other manifestations of the infection, apart from a positive histoplasmin skin test. For this reason no treatment was given

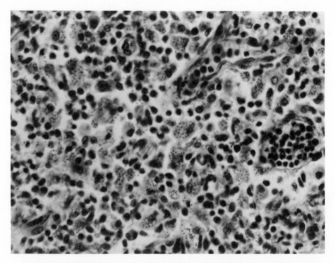

Fig. 26.1.   Even at this magnification the histoplasmas are easily seen in the cytoplasm of the macrophages. The field is from the subepithelial tissue at the margin of the lingual ulcer. As well as the conspicuous accumulation of macrophages there are many lymphocytes and some neutrophils and plasma cells in the exudate.

Haematoxylin–eosin   × 300

at that time. The surgical wound healed well and there has been no recurrence of ulceration.

Three years later (in other words, since publication of the case history in 1961[1]), seeing his dentist for a routine dental check, the patient mentioned that he was feeling run down. The dentist got him to go to his doctor, who recognized that he had Addison's disease. There was no other obvious disorder. Biopsy of an adrenal confirmed the diagnosis of histoplasmosis as the cause of the condition (Figs 26.3 to 26.5).

A course of amphotericin was started: the intravenous dose on successive days was 10 milligrams, 25 milligrams and 50 milligrams. During the third infusion the patient collapsed with acute adrenal cortical insufficiency and almost died. This crisis past, amphotericin therapy was cautiously resumed: the dose was very slowly increased from 1 to 65 milligrams daily and the course then continued over ten weeks, until a total of a little under 4 grams had been given.* Side effects of the antibiotic were not very troublesome (occasional nausea and headache during the infusions, and thrombosis of many of the veins used). Throughout this course the patient was maintained on adrenocortical substitution therapy with cortisone and fludrocortisone: this treatment has been continued ever since. Serial X-ray examination during the course of amphotericin showed the development of calcification in the very large mass of necrotic material that had replaced the adrenal on each side.

There have been no further symptoms of histoplasmosis.

The patient was last seen on his sixty-eighth birthday, in February, 1972. He was in excellent spirits.

Comments

The pathologist who was sent the excised ulcer would even now, eleven years later, probably not be alone in thinking

* Both the daily dose and the total dose of amphotericin given to this patient are about double the level that would nowadays usually be considered appropriate.

the investigation of any but the most commonplace fungal infections to be outwith the competence of the average clinical pathology laboratory. There certainly are cases that may tax an expert mycologist's ability to identify fungi and determine whether they are pathogenic. But most of the pathogens are quite readily identifiable, given commonsense, a good laboratory manual, and basic experience that is well within the capacity of any clinical pathologist to acquire. And when there is doubt there are the experts to whom we may turn for ready help (or whom we might, of course, have asked to do the job from the start, or at least to advise us how to proceed).

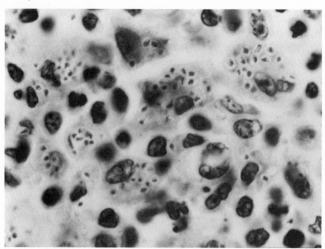

Fig. 26.2A.   A field near the centre of Fig. 26.1, more highly magnified. The appearances of the parasites in the cytoplasm of the macrophages are typical of *Histoplasma capsulatum*. The narrow unstained zone round the cell body of the organism is evident. Because this infection and leishmaniasis tend to be mistaken one for the other, especially in laboratories in parts of the world where neither disease is indigenous,* and therefore where neither is familiar, Fig. 26.2B is included here to show the similarities that account for the occasional confusion.

Haematoxylin–eosin   × 900

---

* To avoid suspicion of chauvinism, the country that I have particularly in mind is best not named. Some of those who, like me, have made the mistake in question will not need to be told where it may happen; others will use their good sense to work it out for themselves.

But it is not just the responsibility of isolating and recognizing fungi that makes some of us shy of them. Through misunderstanding, some pathologists have an exaggerated view of the risks that their staff may be exposed to when fungi

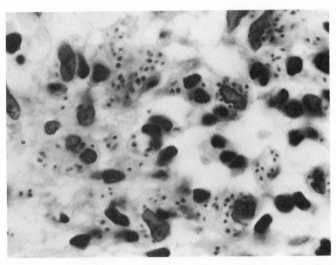

Fig. 26.2B.   This, at the same magnification as Fig. 26.2A and stained in the same way, is a characteristic field from a leishmanial ulcer of a lip, a lesion that could well have been simulated clinically by *Histoplasma capsulatum* infection. The leishmanias (*Leishmania tropica* in this instance) are readily seen in the cytoplasm of the macrophages: it would not be possible in such a preparation to distinguish with certainty between *Leishmania tropica* (the cause of cutaneous leishmaniasis) and *Leishmania donovani* (the cause of visceral leishmaniasis).

Both *Histoplasma capsulatum* and *Leishmania* species are obligate intracellular parasites that infect reticuloendothelial cells almost exclusively. When it is possible to make a direct comparison there is no real difficulty in telling the two organisms apart: but if this comparison cannot be made there is a real possibility of mistaking either for the other. *Histoplasma capsulatum* is larger than the leishmanias, but size alone is often a fallible criterion if there is no opportunity to see the two in succession. Contrary to popular repute, leishmanias are seldom helpfully distinguished by Giemsa or other Romanowsky stains in tissue sections; however, these are very valuable for demonstrating them in films, in which the typical morphology of the parasites is seen at its clearest. The periodic-acid/Schiff and other 'special' stains for fungi react well with histoplasmas but not with leishmanias.

Haematoxylin–eosin   ×900

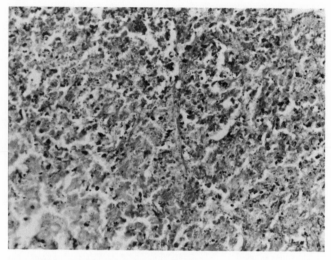

Fig. 26.3.   The patient, perhaps less cooperative than usual because of the unexpected turn of events, insisted on histological proof of the adrenal involvement
before he would agree to treatment. Moreover, he refused to allow any procedure
other than needle biopsy. This was undertaken by a physician experienced in
obtaining renal biopsy specimens, though he tackled the job with little confidence
either in its safety or in the likelihood of its success. In this haematoxylin–eosin
preparation nothing is seen other than necrotic and almost structureless tissue.
See Fig. 26.4.

Haematoxylin–eosin   × 225

are cultured in the laboratory. Such fears thwarted the investigation of the case described in the next chapter. True, some
fungi are highly infective: this is so of *Coccidioides immitis,*
cultures of which on solid media are always in the mould
form and comparatively soon capable of liberating large
numbers of infective spores into the air (see *Memorata,*
Chapter 28). Mycologists do not knowingly deal with coccidioidal cultures except with stringent safeguards. They prefer
that no one work with the coccidioides who has not already
had a primary coccidioidal infection, as shown by a positive
coccidioidin skin test.

The risks from *Histoplasma capsulatum* in the laboratory are
far smaller. For one thing, the histoplasma grows in the in-

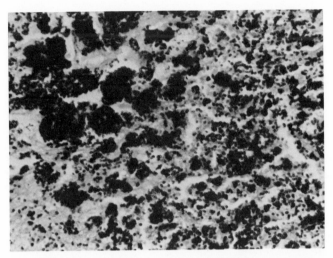

Fig. 26.4. This field in a hexamine–silver preparation corresponds to the haematoxylin–eosin field in Fig. 26.3. The small dark bodies are histoplasmas, still well stained although their failure to show well in the haematoxylin–eosin preparations indicates that they are mostly dead. The particularly compact collections of the fungal cells represent correspondingly heavy parasitization of macrophages. There is no other condition that could present the appearances seen here. See Fig. 26.5 also.

Hexamine–silver   ×225

fective mould phase at room temperature only. The yeast-like phase, which grows at body temperature, is not liable to be carried into the air if the cultures are exposed to draughts, and indeed it is doubtful if the fungus in this form is capable of setting up infection. As cultures are usually grown at 37° centigrade in clinical laboratories, there is little chance of an unexpected isolate of histoplasma proving hazardous.

Histoplasmosis and Addison's Disease. In the USA histoplasmosis is among the commoner causes of Addison's disease, if indeed it is not the commonest. Even so, Addison's disease is extremely rare in comparison with the great numbers of people who have been infected with this mycosis.

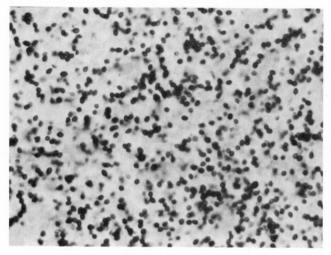

Fig. 26.5.   The higher magnification of this photograph of a field lacking any particularly dense accumulation of the histoplasmas allows the characteristic appearance of the fungal cells to be seen.

Hexamine–silver   × 450

Experience in Britain and elsewhere in recent years has suggested that histoplasmosis contracted in southern or south-eastern Asia is likelier to cause Addison's disease than histo-plasmosis originating in other parts of the world. It is not clear why this should be. I have seen forty-eight patients[3] in Britain or other parts of the north-west of Europe whose histoplasmosis was assumed to have been acquired during long residence in Asia.* The first manifestation in forty-five of the cases was ulceration (often extremely painful) of the mouth, nose, throat, conjunctiva, anus, vulva or penis; none had demonstrable pulmonary involvement (ordinarily, histoplasmosis is a pulmonary infection, and ulceration is an infrequent presentation). Serious symptoms of adrenal in-volvement developed in eighteen of the patients, and eleven

* All forty-eight patients were former European or Australian expatriates who had retired from Asia between one and forty-three years before developing clinical evidence of the infection.

died of this complication. Another remarkable feature was the presence of a peculiar cyst-like form of the fungus in the biopsy specimens from the ulcers (Figs 26.6 and 26.7).

The clinical and pathological findings in such cases beg the question whether there may be a distinct Asian variety of histoplasmosis, counterpart of African histoplasmosis caused by *Histoplasma duboisii* (see Fig. 28.2, page 119) but mycologically related more closely than the latter to the usual form of histoplasmosis caused by *Histoplasma capsulatum*.

Treatment of Histoplasmosis. In the case described in this chapter, and in most of the other forty cases of 'Asian' histoplasmosis

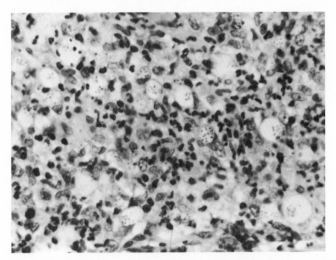

Fig. 26.6.   As well as the usual forms of histoplasma, this field from an oral ulcer includes a score and more of the cyst-like forms of the fungus that may be peculiar to infection acquired in parts of Asia. The appearances are seen more clearly in Fig.26.7.

This patient, an Englishman, had been back in England for five years, after eighteen years of residence in southern Asia, when his infection manifested itself with an ulcer just inside the angle of the mouth.[4]

Reproduced by permission of the Editor of the *American Journal of Clinical Pathology* (the illustration was originally published in the article cited as Reference 4 on page 107).

Haematoxylin–eosin   × 480

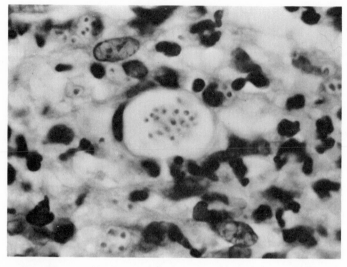

Fig. 26.7.   The cyst-like form of the histoplasma has a distinct fine wall and contains clusters of fungal cells that individually do not differ from cells of *Histoplasma capsulatum* as these are ordinarily seen in tissue sections. This field, which is from the same specimen as Fig. 26.6, also includes several conventional forms of the fungus.

Reproduced by permission of the Editor of the *American Journal of Clinical Pathology* (the illustration was originally published in the article cited as Reference 4 on page 107).

Haematoxylin–eosin   × 950

that I have seen, the patients were treated with amphotericin. Those with painful ulcers were usually relieved of pain within hours of starting treatment, though the ulcers continued to yield viable histoplasmas for up to ten days, and often took several weeks to heal.

The occurrence of acute adrenal cortical insufficiency seemed in some cases to have been precipitated by administration of amphotericin. It is possible that such histoplasma-infected adrenals may become the site of something analogous to the Jarisch–Herxheimer reaction in cases of visceral syphilis when the initial dosage of arsenical drugs or antibiotics has been too high. The presumption is that the sudden death and dissolution of great numbers of the micro-organisms either cause extensive local damage by released 'endotoxins' or trigger an acutely destructive local allergic reaction to these substances. Whatever the mechanism, this complication of 'Asian' histoplasmosis is so grave, carrying a mortality of some thirty per cent, that the very greatest caution is needed in the dosage of whatever antifungal drug is used, and particularly at the start of treatment.

Amphotericin is still* the most widely available drug that is regularly effective against serious histoplasmic infection. Safer, more effective drugs are being developed; some, like 5-fluorocytosine, are already with us, if still under trial. Meantime, amphotericin is often life-saving: yet some physicians deny it to their patients, fearful because of its reputation as a potentially dangerous drug (a fear comparable in its occasional effects to that concerning chloramphenicol—see Chapter 21, page 72).

References

(1) Symmers, W. St C. (1961) Further cases of exotic mycoses seen in Britain—histoplasmosis, chromoblastomycosis, rhinosporidiosis, and phycomycosis. *Transactions of the Royal Society of Tropical Medicine and Hygiene, 55* (June), 201–8.

(2) Earle, J. H. O., Highman, J. H. & Lockey, Eunice (1960) A case of disseminated histoplasmosis. *British Medical Journal, 1* (February 27), 607–11.

(3) Symmers, W. St C. (1972) Histoplasmosis in southern and south-eastern Asia—a syndrome associated with a peculiar tissue form of histoplasma: a study of 48 cases. *Annales de la Société Belge de Médecine Tropicale, 52,* 435–48.

(4) Symmers, W. St C. (1966) Deep-seated fungal infections currently seen in the histopathologic service of a medical school laboratory in Britain. *American Journal of Clinical Pathology, 46* (November), 514–37.

* December 1973.

27 ... and Another ...1

This is a historic case of histoplasmosis, for the patient was the first on record to have acquired histoplasmosis in the British Isles. As *Histoplasma capsulatum* is a fungus that does not occur naturally in these islands, at least up to the time of writing (1973), it is important to note right at the start that the source of his infection is speculative. During the 1939–45 war he entertained many Americans in his home in England, and from time to time they sent him parcels of presents in return for his hospitality. Histoplasmosis is a classic example of a dust-borne inhalational infection. The fungus develops its infective spores only when growing in the saprophytic mould phase, particularly where bird or bat droppings have provided a suitable pabulum. When such dust is disturbed the spores readily take to the air: the severity of a primary infection depends on the number of spores inhaled. There is no evidence that histoplasmosis is conveyed from person to person, so it seems likelier that the Americans' parcels rather than their persons were the source of this man's infection. In other words, his illness is most reasonably explained as an instance of infection by fomites, perhaps packing material that had been contaminated in America (cases of other mycoses probably transmitted in this way are described in *Memorata*, Chapters 30 and 31).

Case

The patient, an entrepreneur, had cut his forehead in a fall on a flinted cliff path in Ireland in 1936: the cut had healed quickly, without stitching. In 1950, when he was 41, the scar became indurated and livid. It was excised: sections showed a silicotic granuloma (Fig. 27.1).*

About six months later the patient noticed that the lymph nodes in his neck, armpits and groins were enlarging. Six months later still he went to his doctor. He was found to have miliary shadowing in his lungs. The Mantoux reaction was weakly positive with 1 in 100 old tuberculin. His serum globulin was 4 grams in 100 millilitres and the albumin–globulin ratio 1·1 : 1. Lymph node biopsy showed sarcoidosis (Fig. 27.2). No treatment was given. He did not have to stop work.

Two and a half years later, in 1954, the patient was without symptom or sign of disease. He gave a strong skin reaction to 1 in 1000 old tuberculin. His serum globulin was 2·6 grams in 100 millilitres and the albumin–globulin ratio 1·8 : 1. The return of the clinical and laboratory findings to normal was interpreted as indicating that his sarcoidosis had regressed spontaneously: he was considered to have recovered.

In 1955 the patient was appointed to an important job in the USA. He had never before been outside the British Isles, even on holiday. Shortly before he heard of this posting he had noticed two small, firm lymph nodes above one clavicle: he considered himself to be otherwise in excellent health. Before leaving Britain, he persuaded his doctor to take out one of the nodes to see if there was any possibility of a recurrence of sarcoidosis: the sections showed a confluent tuberculoid granuloma in which there were very many, very large, multinucleate giant cells (Fig. 27.3). The pathologist was

---

* The formation of sarcoid tissue round and in the vicinity of siliceous foreign matter in the skin was described by a great British pioneer of clinical histology, Samuel George Shattock né Betty (1852–1924), a graduate of University College, London, pathologist to St Thomas's Hospital and for many years curator of the pathological museum of the Royal College of Surgeons of England. The lesion is still sometimes referred to by the name that Shattock gave it, 'pseudotuberculoma silicoticum'; some of its other names are discussed in the account of a classic case (*Memorata*, Chapter 19).

110

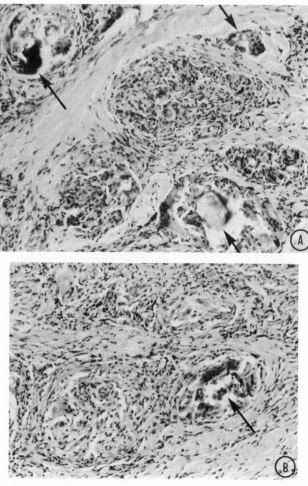

Figs 27.1 A and B. The scar of the injury sustained fourteen years earlier encloses fragments of foreign material (arrowed) round which there is a commonplace proliferation of multinucleate ('foreign body') giant cells—in fact, a characteristic xenosomatogenic polykaryomegalomacrophage reaction, or XPR (see Chapter 22 in *Memorata*). In addition, there is a circumscribed sarcoid type of reaction (better seen in Fig. 27.1 B): this was widespread throughout the scar and its immediate vicinity, but was not related to the visible foreign material in the same intimate way as were the giant cell granulomatous foci. It is this sarcoid response that particularly distinguishes the Shattock granuloma, or 'pseudotuberculoma silicoticum', from an ordinary foreign body reaction (see text).

Microincineration confirmed the siliceous nature of the foreign material in this specimen.

Haematoxylin–eosin   Fig. 27.1 A × 120; Fig. 27.1 B × 145

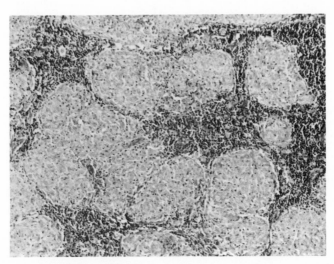

Fig. 27.2.   The patient's first lymph node biopsy showed this picture of pure epithelioid cell aggregates that are not confluent, or that at most merge to an extent that does not completely obscure their separate identity. Multinucleate giant cells, conspicuous in the lymph node examined four years later (Fig. 27.3), are lacking. The appearances are typical of sarcoidosis.

Haematoxylin–eosin   × 80

struck by the differences between the picture of this granuloma and that of the sarcoid lesion of four years before, in which the epithelioid cell aggregates were not so notably confluent and there were no giant cells (Fig. 27.2). He brought the sections to a colleague for a discussion of the significance of the contrast. It was then realized that the giant cells, and some of the mononuclear phagocytes, contained what looked like *Histoplasma capsulatum* (Fig. 27.4). No organisms were found on reviewing the sections of the sarcoid lymph node and of the granuloma in the skin.

Fortunately, the second of the pair of enlarged supraclavicular lymph nodes was still *in situ* and available for culture. It was excised, and a pure growth of *Histoplasma capsulatum* was obtained.

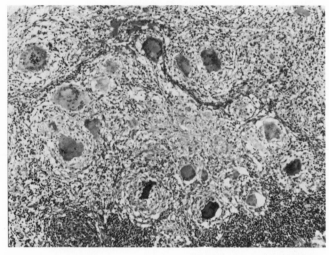

Fig. 27.3. In this lymph node, which became enlarged four years after the biopsy illustrated in Fig. 27.2, there are many very large multinucleate giant cells in the granulomatus tissue: in consequence, the histological picture has a totally different character—and a totally different significance (see Fig. 27.4). As these giant-celled tuberculoid foci fuse they merge so sompletely that in all but the peripheral zone of continuing extension of the reaction they lose the structural outline of their separate origin and identity: this is characteristic of infective granulomas much more than of sarcoidosis.

Haematoxylin–eosin   × 80

It chanced that the laboratory in which these investigations were going on was taken over at the time by another pathologist. When he heard that a histoplasma was being studied there he flew into a rage and had all the cultures and inoculated animals destroyed, believing that his staff had thus been irresponsibly exposed to an intolerable risk.

Meantime, the patient had taken up his work in America. The only investigations that there had been time for before he left were a chest X-ray, which showed nothing abnormal, and a histoplasmin skin test, which was strongly positive. When last heard from, in 1970, he had had no further symptoms of histoplasmosis. He had then been living for fifteen

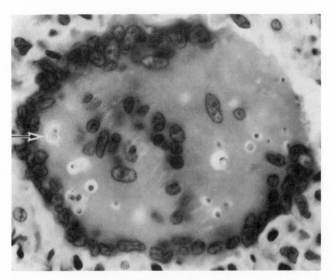

Fig. 27.4.   One of the giant cells in the node illustrated in Fig. 27.3. Most of its nuclei are at the periphery, a few only being scattered in the central mass of cytoplasm. They are unmistakably distinguishable from the histoplasmas, which are considerably smaller and enclosed each in a vacuole-like space that has appeared through shrinkage of the cytoplasm of the host cell during histological preparation of the specimen. The capsule of some of the fungal cells is quite well seen (for instance, at the arrow point).

Since this patient's history was published,[2] specific immunofluorescent staining of sections of the specimen has confirmed that the parasites are *Histoplasma capsulatum* (as had already been shown by the cultures, see text). Proof of the nature of the infection was the more necessary because the histological picture—a multinucleate giant cell granuloma with predominant parasitization of the giant cells—is not typical of histoplasmosis caused by *Histoplasma capsulatum* (compare Figs 27.3 and 27. 4 with Figs 26.1, 26.2A and 28.1, pages 98, 100 and 118).

Haematoxylin–eosin   × 500

years in the eastern central states of the USA : he remarked in his letter that he had long since learnt that no one there, doctors least of all, had the least interest in a case of inactive histoplasmosis.* In contrast, just before leaving Britain, he and his family had been vastly impressed by the descent upon

* A healthy man, whose uncomplicated primary histoplasmic infection was long since, was unlikely to excite interest on this score in an area where the incidence of histoplasmosis is so high that over eighty per cent of the population have been infected.

them and their house and lands of an enthusiastic team of doctors, technicians and medical students, all hunting the histoplasma. The hunt was wholly unsuccessful, indoors and out.

No one else in his household, and none of the numerous domestic fauna, reacted to histoplasmin.

Comment

This case was unusual both clinically and histologically. The primary lesion of histoplasmosis is ordinarily in the lungs: this patient's chest film showed nothing abnormal, either when the diagnosis of histoplasmosis was first made or more recently in America. While it is possible for infection of the supraclavicular lymph nodes with histoplasmosis to be secondary to an intrathoracic focus, as in tuberculosis, such an occurrence is unprecedented as the only clinical manifestation of the infection. The possibility that the infection took place through the skin was considered: no lesion was found, and there was no history of any minor or other penetrating wound that might have given the organism access to the deeper tissues. Again, had the portal of infection been in the upper respiratory tract, or in the mouth or throat, it would hardly have been the lowermost cervical lymph nodes that would have been alone involved when the infection spread from the inoculation site.

Histologically, the strikingly tuberculoid reaction, with uncommonly conspicuous giant cell participation, while by no means inconsistent with histoplasmosis, differed from the more usual histiocytosis.

The unusual features are offset by the demonstration of the fungus in the nodes. Its identity was confirmed by the specialist mycologists in the USA and Europe who vetted the sections and cultures (see also the caption to Fig. 27.4)

The Association with Sarcoidosis. Since this case was first published, in 1956,[1] several colleagues have suggested that the findings that had been interpreted as manifestations of sarcoidosis were in fact due to histoplasmosis. In answer it can be said that the clinical, radiological and histological findings were typical of sarcoidosis, and that no histoplasmas have been found in the original specimens, even on recent re-examination with the help of immunofluorescent methods (fluorescein-labelled anti-*Histoplasma-capsulatum* antiserum). Also, no one has yet shown that the typical picture of sarcoidosis may be a manifestation of histoplasmosis (though, equally, it is impossible to deny that sarcoidosis could, in some instances, be a peculiar response to infection by the histoplasma, just as it is widely thought to be, in some instances, a peculiar response to infection by the tubercle bacillus).

The development of the sarcoid-like granuloma in the scar of the old wound, shortly before the first manifestations of generalized sarcoidosis, is an example of a strange but well-recognized phenomenon. By no means all patients who develop a delayed 'sarcoid' granuloma round foreign bodies prove subsequently to have sarcoidosis: but this sequence is frequent enough for such a reaction to be a warning of what may be in store. The interval between the injury and the appearance of the sarcoid granuloma was fourteen years in this patient's case—it was forty-eight years in the case of a fugitive prisoner of war whose story will be told in Chapter 19 of the last volume of this trio, *Memorata*.

Vandalism. As in the last chapter, we have to note the needless loss of important material because of a pathologist's exaggerated fear about the dangers of dealing with *Histoplasma capsulatum* in the laboratory. Raphael and Schwarz, experienced in the practical study of pathogenic fungi, wrote in 1953, 'Reasonable precautions will . . . protect the laboratory worker against Histoplasma infection'[2] nothing since then has suggested that more than the commonsense and almost universally practised standards of laboratory safeguard is required when working with materials infected by histoplasmas. In contrast, it is life-saving to remember that infinitely more stringent precautions are needed to prevent accidental infection by *Coccidioides immitis,* the cause of coccidioidomycosis: this is a topic that is raised again by the laboratory infections caused by cultures from a case of coccidioidomycosis in Britain, reviewed in Chapter 29 of *Memorata.*

References

(1)   Symmers, W. St C. (1956) Histoplasmosis contracted in Britain—a case of histoplasmic lymphadenitis following clinical recovery from sarcoidosis. *British Medical Journal, 2* (October 6), 786–90.
(2)   Raphael, S. S. & Schwarz, J. (1953) Occupational hazards from fungi causing deep mycoses. *A.M.A. Archives of Industrial Hygiene and Occupational Medicine, 8* (August), 154–65.

28 À Propos *of Histoplasmosis*

(*A Postscript to Chapters 26 and 27*)

After giving a paper at a conference in another English-speaking country, I was asked by the organizing editor to send him the manuscript for early publication in a leading international journal there. The paper summarized cases of histoplasmosis that had been diagnosed in the British Isles. With the exception of the case in the previous chapter (page 108), it was clear that the infections had all been acquired in parts of the world where histoplasmosis is recognized to occur naturally—the relevant geographical circumstances were set out in a separate paragraph in each case summary.

Some months after the manuscript had been posted, a letter came from the editorial secretary of the journal, courteously rejecting the paper in terms that made it sound like the runner-up to the Pullitzer Prize. The salve and balm apart, her letter read:

> Our factuality referee in chief for mycologic content papers indicates histoplasmosis do not occur in England. He animadverts the histoplasmosis diagnosed in error in your MS. cases therefor, relevantly epidemiologic and geopathologic factors of admitability of this diagnosis that is not admitable in connexion the known non occurence of histoplasmosis in the geographic area of your MS. Histoplasmosis in British Hospital Practise Today.

For your greater interest and instruction we are pleased to offer our adviser's further animadvert of your evidence. As for reasons already written the diagnosis histoplasmosis is unacceptable it follows the structures you purport as histoplasma cells in your histologic microphotographs, fig. 1 etc., factually are presumptive *torula* cells, also a fungus that pathologists not familiar

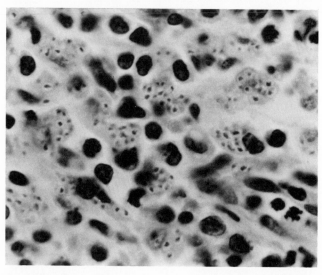

Fig. 28.1.   This figure, illustrating a picture characteristic of histoplasmosis caused by *Histoplasma capsulatum*, is the one that was rejected by a rather famous infective diseasologist who considered it to represent cryptococcosis (see text). Although he practised in a part of the world where histoplasmosis is practically as prevalent as tuberculosis has ever been, he was perhaps less familiar with the microscopical appearances of the fungal infections than with their clinical recognition and treatment.

Pique and bias apart, the picture is typical of histoplasmosis—and *Histoplasma capsulatum* was grown from the same specimen, a laryngeal ulcer. The patient was an elderly man, a lifelong resident of a rural area in Tennessee where histoplasmosis is particularly prevalent, who first lost his voice while on a conducted tour of Blenheim Palace in Oxfordshire, where histoplasmosis does not occur (as it does not occur anywhere in the British Isles). The organisms are significantly smaller even than small-cell strains of *Cryptococcus neoformans* (compare with Fig. 28.2).

Haematoxylin–eosin   × 800

with histoplasmosis mistake with histoplasmosis Darling. Torula disease occurs in your country (refer J.B.M.A. Sept. 1957, Plummer Etal).*

We will accept without precommitment to resubmission the MS. to the factuality advisers with your revise of the indicted comments and torula redesignation of all cases. Hopefully Dr Etal is known to you as he can confirm you the torula identification in your MS. cases.

What was clear after reading the letter was that the journal did not want the paper in its existing form. It certainly sounded

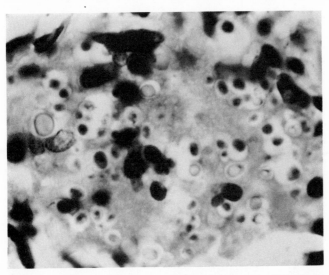

Fig. 28.2. This field is from a cryptococcal ulcer of the skin. The infection was progressing rapidly, and the organisms are smaller than usual and have a less abundant mucous capsule (compare with Fig. 28.3). While the smallest of these cryptococci are no larger than the cells of *Histoplasma capsulatum* in Fig. 28.1, others range in size up to the dimensions of the nuclei of the giant cells that contain them: the histoplasmas, in contrast, are all of the same relatively small order of size. It is *Histoplasma duboisii*, the African histoplasma, that is likely to be confused with these small cryptococci (see Fig. 28.4).

Haematoxylin–eosin   × 800

* Torula (*Torula histolytica*) and torulosis are out-of-date synonyms of cryptococcus (*Cryptococcus neoformans*) and cryptococcosis respectively.

as if the factuality referee had not had time to read the patients' geographical histories and the deduction that their infections had with the one exception been acquired outside the British Isles. 'Fig. 1' of the paper is reproduced here (Fig. 28.1)* and is typical of histoplasmosis (the original caption included a note that *Histoplasma capsulatum* had been cultured from the specimen). Dr Etal was not known to me, but it was possible to trace the reference 'J.B.M.A. Sept. 1957, Plummer Etal'— at least I feel sure it must have been an article by Dr N. S. Plummer *et al.* in the journal of the British Medical Association on 14 September, 1957.†

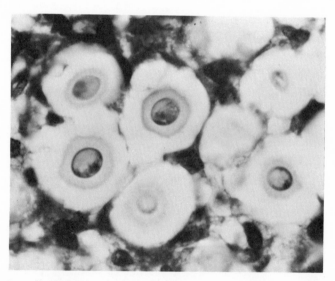

Fig. 28.3.   Typical cryptococci in a slowly growing, clinically silent, pulmonary granuloma—a chance finding in a radiograph of the chest in the course of examination for military service (lobectomy specimen). The fungal cells are much larger and have a much thicker capsule than those illustrated at the same magnification in Fig. 28.2.

Haematoxylin–eosin   × 1000

---

* As the paper was never published the illustration may be shown here without formalities.
† Plummer, N. S., Symmers, W. St C. & Winner, H. I. (1957) Sarcoidosis in identical twins with torulosis as a complication in one case. *British Medical Journal*, 2 (Sep. 14), 599–603.

It happened that I had originally sent the organizing editor of the conference two complete copies of the paper. Embarrassed when he received from the editorial secretary of the journal a copy of her letter to me, on his own initiative he sent the duplicate material to the editor of a rival and equally well known journal. Some months later, the editor of the

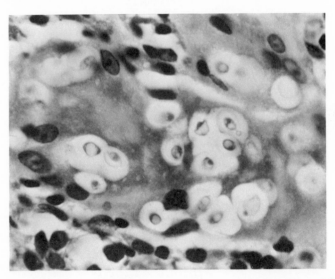

Fig. 28.4.   The well-defined round and ovoid structures are *Histoplasma duboisii* cells. The cytoplasm of the 'foreign body' giant cells has shrunk by artefact, the vacuole-like space attracting attention to the contained fungal cells. The lesion is a granuloma of the skin in a patient, an Irish priest, who spent five weeks on war relief work in Nigeria in 1969, his only visit to Africa. *Histoplasma duboisii* in infected tissues is a much larger cell than *Histoplasma capsulatum* (Fig. 28.1) and can be confused with small forms of cryptococci (Fig. 28.2) and with *Blastomyces dermatitidis*, though seldom excusably. The foreign body giant cell reaction is characteristic of the infections caused by *Histoplasma duboisii*: confusion in interpretation is therefore likeliest when other fungi have caused a conspicuously giant-celled response (as, for instance, in Fig. 28.2).

Histoplasma duboisii is often referred to as 'the African histoplasma', a fair enough designation so long as it does not suggest that *Histoplasma capsulatum*, the usual cause of histoplasmosis, is not part of the African mycological scene. In fact, except in West Africa, most or all cases of histoplasmosis originating in that continent are caused by the latter.

Haematoxylin–eosin   × 800

second journal, who seemed not to know of the paper's fate
at the hands of the other publisher, wrote to me:

> We are expertly informed that your contention that
> histoplasmosis does not occur naturally in your country
> is untrue. Standard reference works on fungus diseases
> (——— 1954, ——— 1962) prove you wrong and we
> look forward to studying your explanation of your
> contrary assertion which had it gone undiscovered was
> calculated to bring grave discredit both to this Journal,
> its editors and publishers and to yourself.
>
> Have you, we wonder, not had the opportunity of
> consulting with mycologists and with physicians expert
> in fungus diseases, particularly pulmonic diseases, in
> England? Such consultation with specialists, sometimes
> with a view to enlisting their collaboration and co-
> authorship, often saves the general author for undeserved
> criticisms.
>
> The authorities cited confirm the views of our own
> special advisers that England is histoplasmosis endemic
> (resp. page 121 and 320). We are surprised that you did
> not pay attention to this fact, the more so as your
> availability of at least one of the works is definitely
> evidenced through your own citation of the book in
> your bibliography. It is a Golden Rule of scientific writing
> never to cite any publication, whether book or periodi-
> cal, without having personally studied it in detail and
> page by page.
>
> If you will correct these inaccuracies and clearly state
> the English origin of the infections in each case we would
> agree to reassess the paper while fully maintaining our
> right to omit or appropriately recast the parts which our
> own special advisers find still needful of omission or
> correction.
>
> Because of the delays already caused by the matters

above commented, it will not be possible for proofs to be sent you as your office is outside the limits of reliable mailing time. Accordingly, and as a gesture of personal good will, we will ourselves attend to proofs on your behalf, and on this occasion without cost to you and in return without accepting any liability for any errors that may escape our vigilance.

The American books that the editor cited—one a manual of clinical mycology and the other a monograph on fungal diseases of the lungs—are misleading in their way of mentioning that cases of histoplasmosis have been reported from 'England' or 'Great Britain'. They failed to consider that the infections could have been picked up in areas geographically remote from these islands.

Another American work—a monograph on histoplasmosis, and no less authoritative than the others—ought to have been as readily accessible to the editorial advisers. It makes precisely this important point that the others overlooked in dealing with the geographical distribution of histoplasmosis:[1]

Finally, human cases of histoplasmosis diagnosed on a histological basis or by culture furnish an insight into the distribution of H. capsulatum. Here the records must be interpreted judiciously, for often an infection has been contracted in areas far from the place of diagnosis. This type of difficulty was illustrated clearly by Symmers when he evaluated the reports of histoplasmosis diagnosed in Britain.

Reference

(1) Ajello, L. (1960) Geographic distribution of Histoplasma capsulatum. In *Histoplasmosis*, edited by H. C. Sweany, pages 88–98. Springfield, Ill.: Charles C Thomas.

29 ... and a Case of Mycoplasmosis?

A young man was killed outright by a car as he ran across a busy road to catch a bus. It was 1946. The cause of death was laceration of the abdominal aorta. Unexpectedly, the forensic pathologist found foci of consolidation up to three or four centimetres across in both lungs, particularly near the hila but also throughout all the lobes.

The pathologist was accompanied by a registrar in training whom he allowed to take parts of the lungs for further examination. Sections showed an interstitial pneumonia with some alveolar exudate. The cells in the pneumonic foci were mostly macrophages and lymphocytes, with few polymorphs. No organisms were found in the sections. The condition was assumed to be a 'primary atypical pneumonia'.

The man's friends were unaware that he had any illness: he had not mentioned any symptoms, though they had noticed that he had had a cough for a week or so. He had gone to work as usual on the day of the accident. There was nothing to suggest that he had been in any way incapacitated by the pneumonia. As clinical illness is characteristically slight in many cases of primary atypical pneumonia, even when there are striking radiological changes in the lungs, such history as was obtained in this case was consistent with the pathologists' diagnosis.

Cultures of material that had been collected from the pulmonary lesions under conditions as nearly aseptic as are possible during any ordinary PM were incubated aerobically on blood agar at 37° centigrade. By the day after the PM a few colonies of pneumococci and *Haemophilus influenzae* had grown. Re-examination of the plates after two days' incubation showed that in addition there were clusters of very small, transparent, colourless colonies, up to a quarter of a millimetre across, though many were scarcely visible even with a hand lens. Under the stereoscopic microscope some of the larger of these colonies had a distinctive appearance, with a tiny, relatively opaque, central elevation surrounded by a broad, flat, transparent areola that had a distinct, delicate edge barely raised above the surface of the medium. The surface of others was completely plane. There was little or no confluence of the colonies that were in contact. Even after incubation for a further couple of days the largest of these peculiar colonies were still no more than half a millimetre across. They consisted of closely packed, very minute, rounded, Gram-negative bodies, staining poorly, not at all clearly distinguishable individually, and seeming to adhere together in clusters.

The bacteriologist to whom the registrar showed the cultures and the minute particles in the films said that these were not organisms—perhaps splash-marks on the medium, artefacts, certainly nothing to waste time on. 'Our job', he said, 'is to recognize pathogens—anything else isn't important in a hospital laboratory.' It can be easy to discourage the stirrings of inquisitiveness in those without an irresistible urge to probe every novel problem. Besides, 'Membership' was on, with a Path. Viva to swot for . . .

Retrospect. Some years afterwards, when the sometime registrar was introduced to the work of Eaton and his colleagues that, in the 1940s, had established the 'Eaton agent' as a cause of primary atypical pneumonia, he wondered if it was possibly this that he had isolated from the pneumonic foci. Eaton's organism—*Mycoplasma pneumoniae,* as it is now named[1]—qualifies today for the attention that the bacteriologist might not have allowed it in his laboratory in 1946. Very possibly, of course, what was grown then was not *Mycoplasma pneumoniae* but one of the mycoplasmas that are easier to culture under such conditions: or maybe it was not a mycoplasma at all but a bacterial L-form (if that is something else). Whatever its identity, its pathogenicity in that case is as dubious today, in retrospect, as it was left undetermined then.

Comment

This was an abortive laboratory study, abandoned prematurely through insufficient curiosity, its potential significance now speculation without importance or value. Maybe its inclusion among the *Curiosa* in these pages will encourage some one who reads it to be less easily deflected when he finds something he doesn't understand and must try to work it out for himself.

Colligation of Chapters 24 to 29

These chapters have dealt with cases of infection by the protozoon *Toxoplasma,* the fungus *Histoplasma* and the *Mycoplasma* (or bacterial L-form?).

Pro-Glossary

The mycoplasmas[1]—the pleuropneumonia group of organisms*—may be stable L-forms of bacteria.

L-forms are bacteria that do not form rigid cell walls. They are thought to be variants, surviving by selection in an

---

* Often casually called PPLO (pleuropneumonia-like organisms) because the first to be recognized was isolated from pleuropneumonia of cattle (in 1898). Can an organism be like pleuropneumonia?

environment that is unsuitable for the corresponding strains that have normal walls. The variants may be stable, or capable of reversion to the normal form. Doctor Emmy Klieneberger-Nobel, who described the L-forms first, in 1935, named them thus because she was working in the *Lister* Institute, in London. L-forms are able to multiply: in this they differ from protoplasts, which are bacterial cells that have lost the rigidity of their cell walls through the actions of lysozymes (enzymes, present in tears and other secretions, that break down the bacterial mucopeptides).

It has been suggested that *Mycoplasma pneumoniae* may be the stable L-form of an α-haemolytic streptococcus, *Streptococcus MG*, because there are agglutinins against this organism in cases of *Mycoplasma pneumoniae* infection.

Reference

(1) Marmion, B. P. (1967) The mycoplasmas—new information on their properties and their pathogenicity for man. In *Recent Advances in Medical Microbiology*, edited by A. P. Waterson, chapter 6, pages 170–253. London: Churchill.

30 Henry Vandyke Carter on Mycetoma or the Fungus Disease of India

A Sequel of Gray's Anatomy

Henry Vandyke Carter was born in Hull on the 22nd of May, 1831. His father, Henry Barlow Carter, and brother, Joseph Newington Carter, were well-known artists: Henry Vandyke, to quote his obituary in the *British Medical Journal*, 'inherited, cultivated, and utilised to good purpose' this family gift. There is a story—it could be apocryphal—that Mrs Carter was so determined that her son Henry should be a great artist that she chose his middle name with this future in mind: the name is reputed to have been mistakenly entered in the parish register as Vandyke by a sexton familiar only with this anglicized spelling of Van Dyck, the form that the baby's mother had intended.

As it turned out, he did not decide on a career primarily in art. Instead, he studied medicine in University College, London, walking the wards of St George's Hospital and in 1852 becoming a Member of the Royal College of Surgeons of England and Licentiate of the Society of Apothecaries. His London MD followed in 1856. When 26, in January, 1858, he joined the Bombay Medical Service as Assistant Surgeon. The rest of his professional life was to be spent in India.

Before leaving London for India, Vandyke Carter had been a demonstrator of anatomy at St George's Hospital. While at St George's he illustrated Henry Gray's *Anatomy* (Fig. 30.1). Robert Howden, editor of the seventeenth to

ANATOMY

DESCRIPTIVE AND SURGICAL.

BY

HENRY GRAY, F.R.S.

FELLOW OF THE ROYAL COLLEGE OF SURGEONS:
AND LECTURER ON ANATOMY AT SAINT GEORGE'S HOSPITAL MEDICAL SCHOOL.

THE DRAWINGS

By H. V. CARTER, M.D.

LATE DEMONSTRATOR OF ANATOMY AT ST. GEORGE'S HOSPITAL.

THE DISSECTIONS

JOINTLY BY THE AUTHOR AND DR. CARTER.

THIRD EDITION,

By T. HOLMES, M.A. CANTAB.

ASSISTANT SURGEON AND LECTURER ON ANATOMY AT ST. GEORGE'S HOSPITAL.

LONDON:
LONGMAN, GREEN, LONGMAN, ROBERTS, AND GREEN.
1864.

Fig. 30.1. Title page of the third edition of *Gray's Anatomy*: 'The Drawings by H. V. Carter, M.D.', edited by Timothy Holmes, MA, FRCS. This was the initial Longmans edition, published by that house in 1864 (the publishers' device is partly obscured in this copy by the encircling library stamp of the Royal Medical and Chirurgical Society). The first edition of 'Gray' was published in 1858,* also in London, by J. H. Parker, who published the second edition in 1860.

Photographed by permission of the Honorary Librarians of the Royal Society of Medicine, London.

* It has proved impossible, so far, to find a copy of the first edition of 'Gray' with the title page intact and with a present owner willing to allow it to be photographed (apart from a colleague in another country who asked for a fee of £104·17, at the then current rate of exchange). Any reader who will fill this gap, without cost to himself but with no compensation for his trouble other than a copy, in due course, of *Exotica*, will be a particularly welcome correspondent.

twenty-third editions of 'Gray', wrote in a biographical note, *Henry Gray, F.R.S., F.R.C.S.*:

> In 1858 Gray published the first edition of his *Anatomy,* which covered 750 pages and contained 363 figures. He had the good fortune to secure the help of his friend, Dr. H. Vandyke Carter, a skilled draughtsman and formerly a demonstrator of anatomy at St. George's Hospital. Carter made the drawings from which the engravings were executed, and the success of the book was, in the first instance, undoubtedly due in no small measure to the excellence of its illustrations.

This was a fair tribute, justly given to one of the great medical illustrators. It is arguable whether the softer, more naturalistic anatomical figures in today's descendants of those original editions* are any better for their purpose than the masterly engravings from Carter's drawings (Fig. 30.2).

Soon after Carter got to India his experience of teaching in London and his association there with Gray led to his being recalled from his duties with the artillery of the Central India Field Force. Instead, he was gazetted to act as professor of anatomy and physiology in the Grant Medical College, then in the process of foundation; he held this office until 1863. At the same time he was attached to the staff of the 'J.J.' (Sir Jamsetjee Jheejeebhoy) Hospital, Bombay, for honorary clinical duties. It was here that he had his introduction to mycetoma, the first of the three diseases that his name was to become particularly associated with, and the one that this chapter is mainly about.†

* Longmans, associated with 'Gray' from 1863, the date of the third edition (the first following Gray's death in 1861, from smallpox, at the age of 34), published the thirty-fifth authorized edition in London in 1973.

† Vandyke Carter's work during the outbreak of 'famine fever' in the late 1870s showed that this disease was the same as the relapsing fever of Europe and caused by the 'spirillum' that Obermeier had found in 1873 to be responsible for the latter. This spirillum is now known as *Borrelia recurrentis,* the borrelia of louse-borne relapsing fever. In India this type of famine fever came to be known as Carter's fever, and the organism was variously

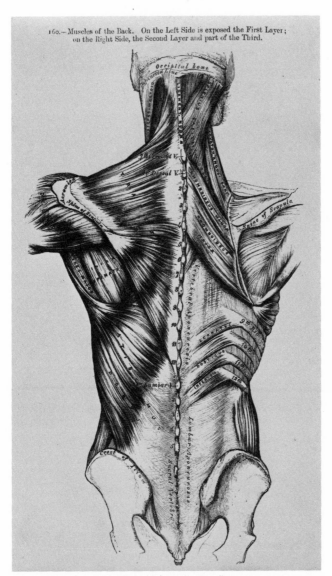

Fig. 30.2. Reproduction of Figure 160 of the third edition of Gray's *Anatomy*— 'Muscles of the Back', an engraving from a drawing by Henry Vandyke Carter. Carter not only made the drawings that illustrated 'Gray' but was responsible for most of the dissections that they were based on.

Photographed by permission of the Honorary Librarians of the Royal Society of Medicine, London.

His work in his earliest years in India was much furthered by the interest and help of a near namesake, Surgeon-Major Henry John Carter, born and buried in Budleigh Salterton (1813–95), of wide scientific interests, a Fellow of the Royal Society, and author of one of the first major studies of the geology of India. Henry John Carter left India in 1862 to settle at home in England. It is not surprising that these two unrelated Henry Carters and their respective achievements, both in medicine and in other fields in India, have been confused by later writers.

Mycetoma, Henry Vandyke Carter's main interest, has been known and recorded in India since ancient times. Its earliest mention in occidental writings was in the *Five Fascicles of the Exotic Politico-Physico-Medical Amenities Collected in Peregrinations Through the Entire Orient,* published in 1712, in Latin, by Engelbert Kaempfer (1651–1716), a peripatetic German doctor from Lemgo in Lippe. Few diseases have so interesting and complex a history (it would be a pleasant exercise to set it down one day—this is not the place). Vandyke Carter's fundamental contributions on mycetoma were three: by 1860 he had recognized that the disease was due to infection by fungi (Figs 30.3 and 30.4); in 1861 he coined the name mycetoma;* and he wrote a monograph,

---

known as *Spirillum carteri* (see below), *Spirochaeta carteri* and, most recently, *Borrelia carteri.*

In 1887, the year before he left India for good, Carter found the organism that causes rat-bite fever, known now as *Spirillum minus*. Rat-bite fever, less common in India than in the Far East, came to be known in India as 'Carter's second fever'.

* Mycetomas are the result of infection either by certain of the true fungi (for example, species of *Madurella*) or by false fungi (particularly species of *Streptomyces* and the actinomycete *Nocardia brasiliensis*: see page 154). They are characterized by chronic suppuration, with the formation of multiple sinuses through the skin and the presence in the exudate of colonies of the fungus ('grains') that usually can be seen with the naked eye.

The name mycetoma is sometimes given, wrongly, to some other manifestations of fungal infections. For instance, some writers still use it of any massive fungal colony occupying a natural or pathological cavity, such as a growth of a candida filling the pelvis of a ureter, or an aspergillus 'fungal ball' (aspergilloma) in an old tuberculous or other cavity in a lung (see page 146). Similarly, solitary mycotic granulomas have also been miscalled mycetomas (for instance, histoplasmomas, coccidioidomycomas and cryptococcomas, to refer to three important varieties by names that are no less inelegant for being used by otherwise respectable international authorities).

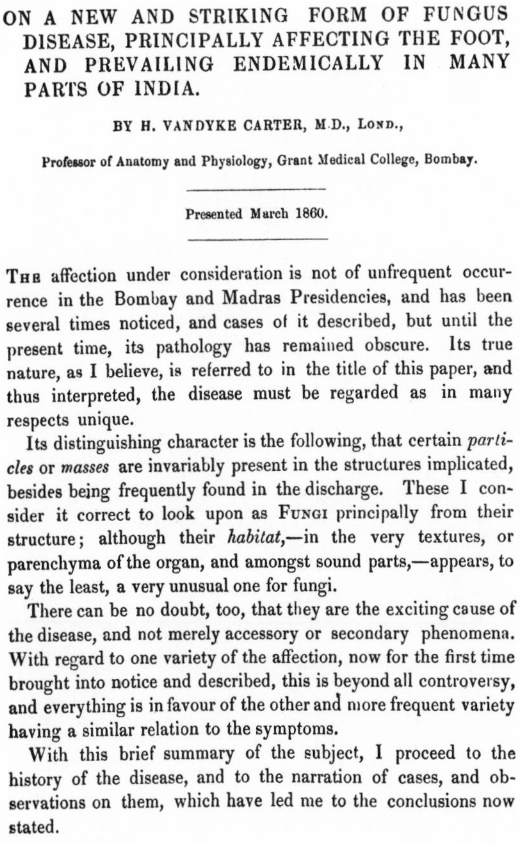

ON A NEW AND STRIKING FORM OF FUNGUS DISEASE, PRINCIPALLY AFFECTING THE FOOT, AND PREVAILING ENDEMICALLY IN MANY PARTS OF INDIA.

BY H. VANDYKE CARTER, M.D., LOND.,

Professor of Anatomy and Physiology, Grant Medical College, Bombay.

Presented March 1860.

THE affection under consideration is not of unfrequent occurrence in the Bombay and Madras Presidencies, and has been several times noticed, and cases of it described, but until the present time, its pathology has remained obscure. Its true nature, as I believe, is referred to in the title of this paper, and thus interpreted, the disease must be regarded as in many respects unique.

Its distinguishing character is the following, that certain *particles* or *masses* are invariably present in the structures implicated, besides being frequently found in the discharge. These I consider it correct to look upon as FUNGI principally from their structure; although their *habitat*,—in the very textures, or parenchyma of the organ, and amongst sound parts,—appears, to say the least, a very unusual one for fungi.

There can be no doubt, too, that they are the exciting cause of the disease, and not merely accessory or secondary phenomena. With regard to one variety of the affection, now for the first time brought into notice and described, this is beyond all controversy, and everything is in favour of the other and more frequent variety having a similar relation to the symptoms.

With this brief summary of the subject, I proceed to the history of the disease, and to the narration of cases, and observations on them, which have led me to the conclusions now stated.

Fig. 30.3. First page of Vandyke Carter's paper reporting his discovery that 'Madura foot' is the result of infection by fungi (*Transactions of the Medical and Physical Society of Bombay*, 1860, N.S. 6, 104–42).

Photographed by permission of the Honorary Librarians of the Royal Society of Medicine, London.

published in 1874, that is a medical classic (Fig. 30.5).[1] His book, it should be needless to add, is magnificently illustrated with coloured lithographs of his own drawings of the specimens (Figs 30.6, 30.7 and 30.11).

134

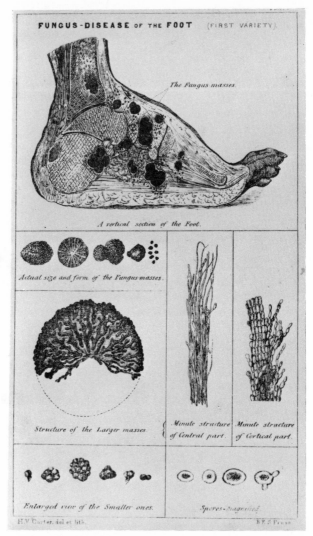

Fig. 30.4.   Reproduction of plate illustrating Vandyke Carter's 1860 paper (see Fig. 30.3). Drawn and lithographed by Carter, it shows an affected foot, bisected, with the dark fungal masses *in situ*. Naked eye and magnified views of these colonies are illustrated to the left of the plate and their microscopical structure to the right. It is clear from the pictures that the appearances are those of infection by a madurella. The foot is apparently the one now in the Royal Army Medical College, Millbank, London, and illustrated in Fig. 30.8 (page 139).

Photographed by permission of the Honorary Librarians of the Royal Society of Medicine, London.

ON

MYCETOMA

OR

THE FUNGUS DISEASE OF INDIA

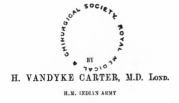

BY

H. VANDYKE CARTER, M.D. Lond.

H.M. INDIAN ARMY

LONDON

J. & A. CHURCHILL, NEW BURLINGTON STREET

1874

Fig. 30.5. Title page of Henry Vandyke Carter's classic monograph *On Mycetoma*, published in 1874.

Photographed by permission of the Honorary Librarians of the Royal Society of Medicine, London.

'Madura foot' is the oldest of the still used synonyms of mycetoma, antedating Carter's introduction of that name by many years, though when it was first used is uncertain. Madura is a town in the Carnatic, about 300 miles to the south-west of Madras. The earliest records of mycetoma in English concern patients attended in the Madura Dispensary by Dr Gill of the Madras Medical Service, whose report was dated 1842. 'Maduramycosis' is a twentieth century coinage. There are at least forty other names, medical or vernacular, but the temptation to remark on even the most picturesque or the most regrettable must be resisted here.

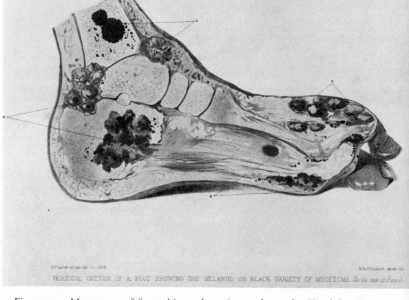

VERTICAL SECTION OF A FOOT SHOWING THE MELANOID OR BLACK VARIETY OF MYCETOMA *See the case at Page 5*

Fig. 30.7.   Mycetoma of foot—bisected specimen, drawn by Vandyke Carter in 1859 (Plate 1 in his monograph *On Mycetoma*). The 'melanoid or black variety' of mycetoma (*Madurella* infection): the dark colonial masses are in cavities in the swollen soft tissues and in the bones.

Photographed by permission of the Honorary Librarians of the Royal Society of Medicine, London.

Vandyke Carter's accounts make it clear that he recognized the fungal nature of the disease from microscopical examination of the colonial grains. He described 'melanoid' and 'ochroid' mycetomas, the first with black or dark brown fungal colonies and the second with pale colonies: we should now recognize these respectively as madurellae and streptomycetes.

Although he referred to one experiment that resulted in the growth of a brown mould, conceivably a madurella, it was a pink mould isolated from other cases that he thought to be the cause of the disease. He sent cultures of the latter to England for identification by the Reverend Mr Berkeley, of Wansford, near Peterborough, an eminent naturalist who deserves to be recognized as one of the first mycologists. The other 'Carter of India', Henry John, then recently returned to England, assisted Mr Berkeley in his investigations. The latter, therefore, intending 'to record the labours of the two Carters, united in their love of science though not in consanguinity', gave the name Chionyphe carteri to this supposed cause of 'the fungus foot of India'. In fact, it was undoubtedly a saprophytic contaminant of the amputation specimens.

That was in 1862. It was not until 1894 that any of the causal organisms of mycetomas was isolated and identified in cultures: Jean Hyacinthe Vincent, a French army doctor, and, a few weeks later, Rubert William Boyce, in University College in London, each isolated a 'streptothrix' (streptomyces, in today's terms), the former from a specimen examined in Algeria and the latter in one from India. A madurella, though one had possibly been grown by Henry Vandyke Carter 36 years earlier, was first isolated with certainty in 1898, by James Homer Wright in the Massachusetts General Hospital, Boston.

A chest complaint of several years' standing obliged Vandyke Carter to retire from the Indian Medical Service in

1888. This was the price of thirty years of unrelaxing involvement in medical practice, research, teaching and administration in India, often under difficult climatic and professional conditions. He had never sought honours. His work was acknowledged, two years after his retirement, by his appointment as one of the Queen's honorary physicians, with the rank of Deputy Surgeon-General, on the retired list. He died of his lung trouble at his home in Scarborough on the 4th of May, 1897, a few days short of his sixty-sixth birthday.

A Hundred Years On: A Search for Original Vandyke Carter Specimens

At various times, when on furlough or in response to requests addressed to him in India, Vandyke Carter presented specimens of mycetoma to medical museums in the United Kingom. In 1962, just over a century after his first publications on mycetoma, I was able with the patient help of their curators, to arrange a search for these specimens in all the museums that might conceivably be their present quarters. It resulted in reviewing a number of old mycetomas, but only one that he had described turned up among them. This was in the pathological collection in the Royal Army Medical College on the Millbank in London (Fig. 30.8). Thanks to the enthusiastic help of Colonel (now Major-General) H. C. Jeffrey, late the Royal Army Medical Corps, and Dr Seymour J. R. Reynolds of Charing Cross Hospital, I was able to have this specimen X-rayed (Fig. 30.9): I wonder if Vandyke Carter, who died in 1897, two years after Röntgen's discovery, ever saw a 'skiagraph' of a mycetoma.

Histological examination of a block of tissue that Dr Jeffrey allowed me to take from the specimen in 1962 showed unexpectedly good stainability, in spite of almost a century in goodness knows what varieties of preserving fluids. Fig. 30.10

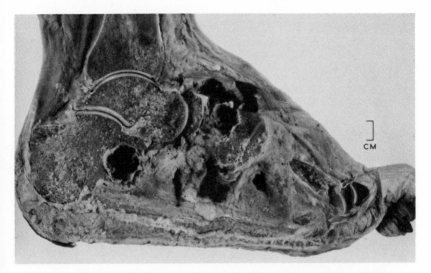

Fig. 30.8.   One of Vandyke Carter's specimens of mycetoma, photographed in 1962 while on loan from the pathological collection of the Royal Army Medical College, Millbank, London, by courtesy of Colonel (now Major-General) H. C. Jeffrey, late the Royal Army Medical Corps. The photograph may be compared with the lithograph of the drawing reproduced in Fig. 30.4 (page 134). The fungal colonies—the black masses in the photograph—appeared black or very dark brown in the preserved specimen. Fig. 30.9 is a radiograph of the specimen and Fig. 30.10 a photomicrograph. (*Photograph by Miss P. M. Turnbull*)

illustrates part of one of the fungal colonies in the granuloma —it is unmistakably a madurella.

Another Original Vandyke Carter Specimen[2]

One of the illustrations in Carter's book shows a mycetoma of a hand (Fig. 30.11). Because involvement of the hand is comparatively rare,* I was especially keen to trace any such

---

* The feet are affected by mycetoma so much oftener than other parts because they are particularly exposed to wounding by thorns and the like that carry the fungi responsible for the infection. Three factors contributing to the occurrence of mycetomas are: (*a*) a climate that supports the saprophytic existence of these fungi in soil; (*b*) spiny or thorny shrubs that, carrying the organism, can introduce it into the tissues when they pierce the skin; and (*c*) a barefoot way of life. Similar factors have their part in the causation of two other important fungal infections—sporotrichosis (page 161) and cutaneous chromomycosis (chapter 8 in *Exotica*).

specimen extant from Carter's experience. None of the few manual mycetomas that the enquiries in 1962 had brought to light could possibly have had any connexion with him, and this particular quest seemed unsuccessful.

Some time later, on my way to work and held up for an hour in an Underground train, stopped in a tunnel by a signal failure, I passed the time checking from memory the possible locations of Carter mycetomas. After listing all the medical museums in these islands that I could think of, it was suddenly obvious that there was one that I had not written to—the Pathology Museum of Charing Cross Hospital Medical School, in London, of which at the time I was curator. An hour or so later, the hand that Carter's lithograph showed was on my bench. Macerated and imperfect, and therefore

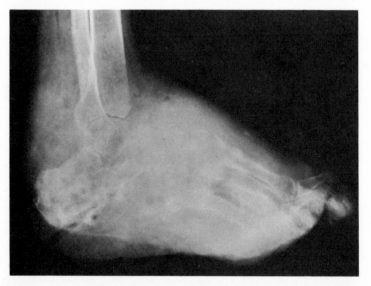

Fig. 30.9.   X-ray picture of the specimen in Fig. 30.8. The extent of the destruction of the bones of the instep and the rounded cavities formed by the fungal colonies in other bones (particularly the calcaneus) are well shown.

Radiograph prepared in 1962 by courtesy of Dr Seymour J. R. Reynolds, Charing Cross Hospital, London. (*Photographic copy by Miss P. M. Turnbull*)

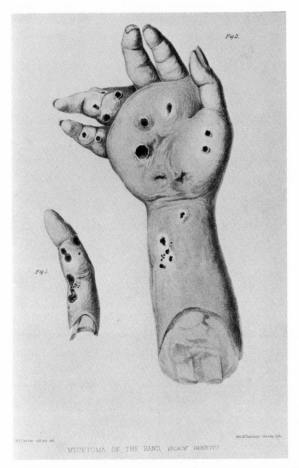

Fig. 30.11. Mycetoma of hand and mycetoma of a finger, drawn by Vandyke Carter 'from nature' (Plate 3 in his monograph *On Mycetoma*). He referred to it as the 'black variety'—as we should say, caused by a madurella. The drawing of the hand appears to be of the specimen that is illustrated in Fig. 30.12.

Photographed by permission of the Honorary Librarians of the Royal Society of Medicine, London.

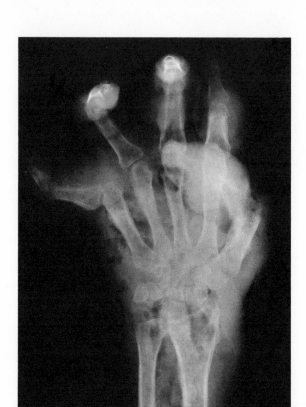

Fig. 30.12.   Radiograph of a mycetoma of a hand—a specimen given by Vandyke Carter to Charing Cross Hospital in 1873, and apparently that shown in his drawing reproduced in Fig. 30.11. The X-ray picture was made in 1963 by courtesy of Dr Seymour J. R. Reynolds, Charing Cross Hospital, London. The bones show marked periosteal reaction but no excavation (compare with Fig. 30.9); the areas of radiolucency are artefacts in the soft tissues, in places superimposed on the bones. The prominence of the periosteal changes is more characteristic of streptomycosis than madurellosis. The lack of evident deeper involvement of bone is unexpected in the presence of such large colonial masses in the soft tissues (see Fig. 30.11). (*Photographic copy by Miss P. M. Turnbull*)

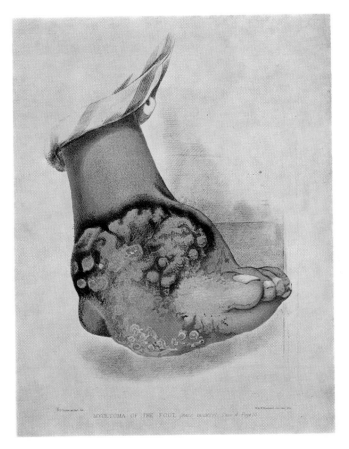

Fig. 30.6. Mycetoma of foot, drawn by Vandyke Carter 'from
nature' (Plate 5 in his monograph *On Mycetoma*). The deformity of the
foot is characteristic: inflammatory swelling of the soft tissues has
filled the hollow of the sole and formed a rounded mass over the
instep. The raw openings of numerous sinuses are seen, and cicat-
rization of others has been accompanied by patchy changes in pigmentation.

The original caption described this as the 'pale variety' of mycetoma—that is, mycetoma caused by a fungus that forms pale
('ochroid') colonial masses in the tissues: in India, such a fungus is
likely to be a species of streptomyces.

Photographed by permission of the Honorary Librarians of the
Royal Society of Medicine, London.

From an 'Agfacolor' transparency (same size)

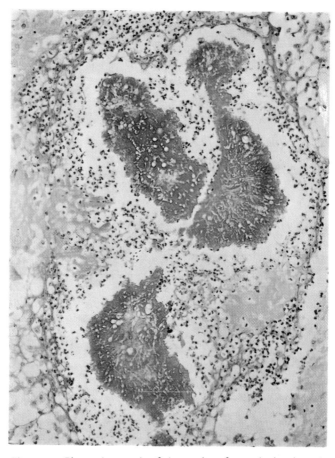

Fig. 30.10. Photomicrograph of tissue taken for sectioning in 1962 from the Vandyke Carter specimen illustrated in Figs 30.4, 30.8 and 30.9. The preservation is so unexpectedly good that, with skill and patience, my colleague Mr F. D. Humberstone was able to produce perfectly stained sections. The position of the hyphae and vesicle-like 'chlamydospores' of the fungus is clearly indicated by the pale areas within the fragments of the colony. These fungal elements are often outlined by a dense brown zone that merges into the paler brown or eosinophile homogeneous substance that forms the bulk of the colonial structure. The brown colour is due to the natural pigmentation of this 'cement': it accounts for the dark brown or black appearance of the colonial masses when seen with the naked eye (see Fig. 30. 8). The thin fibrinopurulent exudate seen in the photograph was contained within the sinus lined by granulation tissue in which these colonial fragments lay.

Haematoxylin–eosin × 160 *From an 'Agfachrome' transparency*
(same size)

long cupboarded out of sight, it was recorded in an ancient 'Accessions Book':

> 'Received of Surgeon-Major H. V. Carter, 1873 : in spirituous *Liquor Conserv.,* a fungus hand from India (the same *delin.* H. V. C. in a Plate to his *op.* "On the Mycetoma", presently setting in London).'

The specimen is no longer suitable for illustration other than as in Fig. 30.12.

References

(1)   Carter, H. V. (1874) *On Mycetoma or the Fungus Disease of India.* London: Churchill.
(2)   Symmers, W. St C. (1970) Curiosa et exotica. *British Medical Journal,* 4 (December 26), 763–7 [Presidential Address, Section of Pathology of the Royal Society of Medicine, London, session 1969–70].

31 Madura Foot (Mycetoma Pedis) of the Hand

There was, in an Irish museum, a specimen that bore this label.*

---

* In a London museum there is a specimen labelled 'Turban Tumour of the Foot'—a diffuse form of sweat gland adenomatosis that ordinarily occurs only in the scalp, its appearances there being for some reason likened to a turban.

32 A Case of Camembert

A woman of 50 or so had been living in Normandy for twenty-five years when she had a small haemoptysis. There were no other symptoms. She and her husband ran a small cheese-dairy, making mainly Camembert cheese. The doctors who examined her noted that her breath had a distinctly caseous smell, reminding them of Camembert that has gone slightly rancid.

The X-rays showed a cavity in the upper lobe of one lung, with appearances typical of a fungal ball free within the cavity. The films have since been—er—'lost' (lost, at any rate, to those legitimately entitled to them), but the picture was essentially the same as in Fig. 32.1. No fungal elements were found in the sputum.

The involved lobe was removed. The origin of the cavity could not be recognized. Its tough fibrous wall was partly lined by stratified squamous epithelium that elsewhere had been eroded, exposing hyperaemic granulation tissue, presumably the source of the bleeding. The cavity contained a densely matted, ball-like colony of a penicillium, and not, as had been expected, an aspergillus (see Fig. 32.1, caption).

After the operation the patient was chesty and her treatment included a series of penicillin injections. On the day after starting penicillin she developed an itchy rash that subsided when the drug was stopped, and reappeared and again subsided when a different preparation of penicillin was given and, because of the rash, withdrawn. Skin tests showed marked sensitivity to penicillin, although she had never been

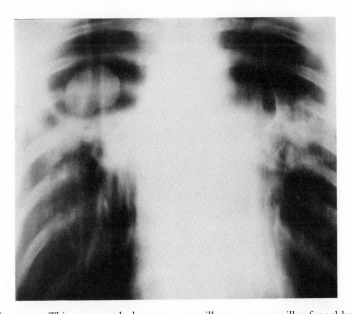

Fig. 32.1. This tomograph shows an aspergilloma, an aspergillus fungal ball, lying free in a cavity in the apical part of the right lung. Such intracavitary colonies can grow very quickly, often eventually filling the space so that only a narrow air zone is demonstrable between the ball and the wall of the cavity. The cavity may be tuberculous in origin, or due to sarcoidosis, bronchiectasis, chronic lung abscess, congenital cyst or emphysematous bulla. The fungus responsible is usually a species of aspergillus; rarely, other organisms have been identified—the penicillium in the case described in the text of this chapter, and in other cases *Allescheria boydii* (a fungus more familiar as a cause of mycetomas of the 'Madura foot' type).

Illustration provided by Dr N. S. Plummer, Charing Cross Hospital.
(*Photographic copy by Miss. P. M. Turnbull*)

treated with penicillin before the lobectomy and the drug had not been in use on the farm. She had no history of other manifestations of allergy. It was suggested that the penicillium in her lung might have sensitized her, perhaps through producing penicillin itself, but it seems improbable that this was more than a fancy. There was no evidence of penicillin production by the fungus isolated *in vitro* from the operation specimen.

The mycologists who studied her fungus identified it as a somewhat unusual strain of *Penicillium camembertii*, one of the moulds concerned in the production of Camembert and some other cheeses. It is not a species recognized to be potentially pathogenic—but, indeed, there are scarcely any acceptable cases of any form of infection in man or animals caused by penicillia.

Comment

Aspergillomas and other intracavitary fungal masses, such as the penicillioma mentioned above, are still sometimes referred to as mycetomas. This term is better reserved for fungal diseases of the 'Madura foot' type, the subject of Chapters 30 and 31 in this book (see footnote on page 131). If this seems a pedantic restriction, perhaps it may be more acceptable if one remembers that the intracavitary fungal ball is really outside the body, in the sense that it lies in the lumen of the cavity and that there is no fungal invasion of the tissues themselves, no mycotic granuloma, at least under natural conditions. Invasion of the lung is a rare development, resulting from resistance being lowered by side effects of corticosteroids, cytotoxic drugs and the like, given in treatment of some other disease: its occurrence is an instance of what has been called 'opportunistic' infection (see page 76).

Reference

(1)   Symmers, W. St C. (1958) In *Sensitivity Reactions to Drugs—A Symposium organized by the Council for International Organizations of Medical Sciences,* edited by M. L. Rosenheim, R. Moulton, S. Moeschlin and W. St C. Symmers, page 115. Oxford: Blackwell Scientific.

33 'It Wasn't the Wine . . . It Was the Salmon'*

The Case of the Navel Boil

A young lady, served with smoked Scotch salmon at her first royally formal dinner, found a bone of the fish in her mouth, too sharp and long to swallow safely. As wife of the guest of honour she sat on her host's right and all the time in view of the television cameras. Anxious not to embarrass her hostess, her husband or herself, she tried to manoeuvre the bone discreetly away, but, as happens on these occasions, it stuck momentarily to her lip, then fell inside the bodice of her dress. Home and at ease again at the end of the evening, the bone proved to have disappeared. She was not concerned, for there seemed an obvious explanation.

About two years later, when she was pregnant, she was examined by an obstetrician. He chanced on a tender point two centimetres or so below the umbilicus and a little to one side. His patient had not previously been aware of this sore spot, but from then on she formed the habit of pressing it with her finger-tips. A few weeks later she drew the doctor's attention to a short, firm ridge that could just be felt under the skin in the painful area—he said it was a thrombosed vein and of no importance.

Nine months passed, and then, well after her confinement, she began to suffer a constant ache in the abdominal wall in

* Charles Dickens: *Pickwick Papers*.

147

the vicinity of the umbilicus. The earlier tenderness had become less marked and less localized and the 'thrombosed vein' could no longer be felt. The aching soon became severer and her doctor could feel a thickening of the tissues immediately below and to the right of the umbilicus. Shortly afterwards the patient complained that her umbilicus had become itchy—a little seropurulent discharge was seen coming from one of its lower skin folds. A surgeon was called in and decided to explore the abdomen, considering it possible that there might be an umbilical sinus or fistula related to persistence of the vitelline duct.

The laparotomy showed nothing abnormal within the peritoneal cavity. There was an ill-defined mass of scar tissue in the subcutaneous fat near the umbilicus and corresponding to the thickening that had been felt clinically. The scar was dissected out and sent to the laboratory. The first sections showed a chronic non-specific inflammatory infiltrate in dense fibrotic tissue. Because there was no clue to the cause of the scar the rest of the specimen was carefully sliced: this disclosed a pointed fish bone, almost three centimetres long, buried in the fibrotic mass. A fibrous tract ran toward the umbilicus from the scar. There was a little suppuration round the bone and in minute foci along the tract: this probably accounted for the discharge from the umbilicus. No organisms were seen in the sections. There was no umbilical discharge after the operation.

Comment

The only likely explanation of the presence of the fish bone in the subcutaneous tissue is that it lodged in the umbilicus during the evening of the dinner and worked its way through the skin. This could happen painlessly, for the depths of the umbilicus are relatively insensitive in some people. It must surely have been the bone that was felt through the skin during her pregnancy, not a thrombosed vein, which would have been as unusual in this situation as the foreign body.

Swallowed bones are well known to be able to pierce the wall of the stomach or bowel and enter the peritoneal cavity or lodge in adjacent structures. This may lead to general peritonitis, but oftener a localized inflammatory mass develops round the bone, either in the abdominal cavity or in the tissues of the abdominal wall.[1] The granulomas that develop in the latter situation are usually just outside the peritoneum, but sometimes the bone migrates to the subcutaneous tissue, and may even point through the skin and so discharge itself. In the case of the embarrassed dinner guest, the absence of anything abnormal within the abdomen favours the view that the bone must have entered by the navel channel.

Reference

(1)   Gunn, A. (1966) Intestinal perforation due to swallowed fish or meat bone. *Lancet, i* (15 January), 125–8.

34 Tumbu the Man-Eater

The Case of the Naval Boil

A naval officer taking passage in a troopship from the UK to Egypt round the Cape in 1941 was luckier than most of his fellow passengers in being allowed to spend a few hours ashore in Freetown, Sierra Leone, a welcome diversion after dull weeks out of the Clyde without a break in the frustrating monotony of being a sailor at sea as a passenger. The ship stayed only a few days, just enough for the convoy to take on provisions, water and fuel. About ten days after putting back to sea the officer came to the sick bay because of a 'boil' on one arm, near the shoulder.

The boil seemed to be on the point of bursting, its pale core raising the still intact but paper-thin epidermal covering. The medical officer gently stretched the skin until the epithelium over the cavity tore and a little bloody serum escaped. Looking at the small hole that had resulted he was startled to see a sinuously moving whitish body, apparently filling the cavity. A little careful pressure then delivered the thing on to the surface of the skin: there it rested a few moments motionless, and then—seemingly as the result of a sudden curving contraction—fell to the deck, where it lay briefly relaxed before moving steadily, if sluggishly, toward the dark, undeterred by obstacles put in its way.

Carefully retrieved, the creature was seen to be a bot, or maggot, about a centimetre long and a third as much across

the thickest of its dozen or so body segments (see Fig. 34.1).
The MO's fiancée had given him, for this first excursion into
the tropics, a copy of *Manson's Tropical Diseases*. The answer
to the mystery was, of course, in the pages of that abundant
work—his patient had succoured a larva of the tumbu fly,
tumbu the man-eater, *Cordylobia anthropophaga,** and
brought the doctor his first acquaintance with human myiasis.[1] Somewhere in Freetown the patient must have come the
way of a predatory larva, newly hatched from an egg laid on
the ground and actively crawling in search of a friendly skin
to burrow into.

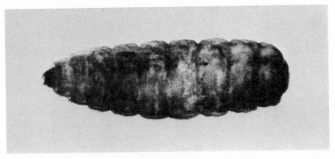

Fig. 34.1.   Larva of *Cordylobia anthropophaga,* the tumbu fly, from another case
(one of those peripatetic external examiners).

× 5

The 'boil' healed quickly. The larva died, in spite of the
MO's efforts to rear it—efforts that left him with an unfading
reminder of the occasion in the form of a blue tattoo in the
skin of the left thumb, where traces of rust from a war-
economy triangular needle marked the site of a blood-letting
in the endeavour to find some nutriment acceptable to the
animal. Thinking back, I fear it died of cosseting.

* Cordylobia it is, c-o-r-d-y-l-o-b-i-a, though medical editors everywhere, schooled on
  condyles and condylomas, will miscorrect it to condylobia, which it isn't.

Comment

In this first meeting with a tumbu larva the ship's doctor was lucky to have to deal with one ripe and ready to emerge from its pit in the patient's skin. Later he was to learn how tenaciously these creatures can dig their spiracles into the tissues, resisting any effort to extract them, short of disintegration— and disintegration resulted all too often in the spiracle remaining firmly attached, when a thoroughly unpleasant and persistent inflammatory reaction was the usual effect. Patients, testy flag officers in particular, were liable to blame this outcome on the MO's incompetence, rightly—if incompetence and inexperience are the same.

Still later the MO learnt the simple (though not always successful) trick of pouring water over the hole in the infested skin, which should asphyxiate the larva, causing it to separate its anchoring spiracles and yield to compression. Another manoeuvre, known in some military medical circles as the RSPCA treatment, or antivivisection (or Home Office) produre, entailed parenteral administration of chloroform to the larva before its expedited extraction by the application of forceps. Whatever the effects on the parasite, the local effects on the host of the chloroform that inevitably escaped into the cavity of the boil caused the anaesthetist to come in for some criticism. From personal experience it is understandable why this should have been so.

Indigenous Bot Boils in Britain. As an epilogue to this history, a case of myiasis in London is a reminder that such lesions are not all tropical exotica. The patient was a young down-and-out (not a drug addict), admitted with acute tuberculous pneumonia from which he died within the week. On admission his clothing and his person were dirty with the filth and stench of months of neglect. He was flea-ridden and infested by head, body and crab lice. He had septic scabies, and syphilis and chronic gonorrhoea. And all over his body there were boils and small ulcers from which larvae of *Musca domestica,* the common house fly, emerged in their hundreds.

A somewhat similar case in Glasgow confirms that such neglect is possible in this age in these islands.[2]

Exotic Bot Boils in Britain. And, as a postscript, a mention of a tumbu larva emerging from the neck of one of the extern examiners (see page 72), who, after a pleasant and not too busy stint in a West African university, flew home to London and there hatched out his larva (Fig. 34.1), much to his horrified disgust, for he was a cleanly man and did not understand how such a thing could have happened to him.

References

(1) Wilcocks, C. & Manson-Bahr, P. E. C. (1972) *Manson's Tropical Diseases,* 17th edition, pages 1118–25. London: Baillière Tindall.
(2) Logan, J. C. P. & Walkey, M. (1964) A case of endemic cutaneous myiasis. *British Journal of Dermatology, 76* (May), 218–22.

35 Brazilian 'Boils'[1]

A Brazilian student living in London went to a general practitioner because of what he took to be a crop of persistent boils over the back of one shoulder. They had started to appear before he left Brazil several weeks previously and had been slowly increasing in size and number. The doctor agreed that they were boils. In the course of six months he tried one antibiotic after another with no more than slight and transitory improvement. The lesions continued to discharge thin pus and, as they involved a wider and wider area about the shoulder, caused the patient increasing discomfort and embarrassment.

One day he met a fellow South American, a Venezuelan doctor on a postgraduate course in Britain. As soon as the Venezuelan saw the lesions he recognized the condition to be a mycetoma. On his advice the patient went to another British doctor, who confessed himself out of his depth and arranged for consultation with a surgeon. The 'boils' proved to be sinuses, and in the exudate from one of them small fungal 'grains' were found. Cultures confirmed the Venezuelan doctor's forecast that the organism would prove to be the actinomycete, *Nocardia brasiliensis*. There was no radiological evidence of involvement of the bones.

Treatment with a long-acting sulphonamide, sulphamethoxypyridazine, resulted in steady improvement and eventual cure.

Comment

This patient was fortunate that his mycetoma, in spite of its long duration, had not spread into the underlying bones. Mycetomas in less characteristic sites, such as his, share with the classic forms ('Madura foot' is the type example; see page 136) a natural tendency to extend from the soft tissues into the bones. Once bone is infected the disease is much more difficult to eradicate.

Nocardia brasiliensis has a distribution far wider than its name suggests. As well as being the commonest cause of mycetomas in many parts of South and Central America it is prevalent in Mexico and in much of West Africa. It is almost alone among the organisms causing mycetoma in its sensitivity to drugs that can be administered reasonably safely over the long periods that are required for cure, particularly in the presence of skeletal involvement. These drugs are the sulphones, particularly dapsone, and the long-acting sulphonamides: their use has given cases of nocardial mycetoma an outlook vastly better than those caused by other organisms.[2]

The related aerobic actinomycete, *Nocardia asteroides,* an organism of worldwide distribution, is not a cause of mycetoma, except possibly in very exceptional cases. In contrast, it is responsible for visceral suppuration, particularly pneumonia and brain abscess, and usually as an 'opportunistic' infection (but see page 22).

Grievance. The delay in diagnosing this Brazilian visitor's infection is just one instance of the commonplace failure to consider the possible significance of patients' geographical histories. Bearing in mind that knowing where his patient has been in the world is helpful to the doctor only if he knows what diseases he should therefore be on the look-out for . . .

References

(1) Symmers, W. St C. (1966) Deep-seated fungal infections currently seen in the histopathologic service of a medical school laboratory in Britain. *American Journal of Clinical Pathology, 46* (November), 514–37. [Case 30: The patient was Brazilian, not Venezuelan as stated in the case summary.]

(2) Cockshott, W. P. & Rankin, A. M. (1960) Medical treatment of mycetoma. *Lancet, 2* (November 19), 1112–4.

36 As Gáirdin Rós i gCualain*

or The Party Piece[1]

'But ne'er the rose without the thorn'
(Herrick, *The Rose*)

A pathologist was unwillingly at a sherry party in London. Edging away from the noise he gained a corner of the room where a Paul Henry on the wall had caught his envious eye. His interest satisfied for the moment, he then realized that he had put himself into the sort of strategically foolish position that the more experienced party man would never be in, with no escape route from an enclosed position. The wall was behind him, on his right a beautiful Broadwood fortepiano of 1822 and on his left a not far short of life-size mid twentieth century marble replica of the Capitoline Venus. Too late he saw his way covered by his kind, but not always tactful, hostess, bearing down with the clear intention of introducing him to a somewhat sickly-looking young man whom she had in tow.

---

* *As Gáirdin Rós i gCualain*: A rose garden in County Dublin. Irish calligraphy by Captain Kevin Danaher, Irish Folklore Commission.

'My dear doctor', she said, knowing both his disinclination for shop on social occasions and just how to overcome it, 'You will please me so much if you will allow me to present to you Mr———: he has a story to tell you, and I know it will interest you to hear it . . .'

Who goes to sherry parties to listen to strangers' medical autobiographies? It certainly isn't doctors, and least of all those not in practice. But the pathologist's reluctance was quickly overcome by the young man himself. A student of laws, he also had all the natural ease with language, and the charm and wit, that for generations had marked his family of Irish men of letters. He began his story at its beginning, and from the beginning the pathologist forgot his vexation.

Three years before, on his twenty-first birthday, the student had torn the skin of the inner edge of his right hand on a thorn while pruning rose bushes in his mother's garden in County Dublin. The wound, though all of three centimetres long, was no more than skin deep, except at the end where the thorn had dug well into the tissues. After a few days the scratch began to fester and the tissues about it became indurated. By the end of a week the wound had become a linear ulcer, with bright red floor and soft, slightly undermined, purplish margin that bled easily when touched. The ulcer enlarged slowly and three or four small nodules appeared in the skin between it and the wrist. One of these nodules became an ulcer like that at the site of the wound; the rest disappeared.

During nine months following the injury a succession of nodules formed in the subcutaneous tissue along the line of the lymphatic vessels of the back and the inner aspect of the forearm, in the antecubital fossa and for a short way above the elbow on the inner side of the arm. The nodules mostly broke down, discharging a little blood-stained matter and becoming transformed into chronic ulcers. There was con-siderable induration of the tissues between the ulcers, The patient had little or no pain or physical discomfort. He lost a good seven kilograms in weight during the first year or so of the illness; after that his weight kept steady, and his general health was little disturbed. By the end of the first year the disease had reached its greatest extent: there was little change in the lesions during the following two years, apart from a tendency to heal over, with some scarring, and then break down again. From time to time he noticed transient enlargement of lymph nodes in the axilla of the affected side.

The student was working in England during these three years and saw a succession of doctors. Various diagnoses were suggested, including syphilis, tuberculosis, farcy (glanders), angiosarcoma, malignant melanoma and mycosis fungoides. One surgeon had told him that he was a 'sadomasochistic psycopath' and accused him of producing the lesions by stubbing lighted cigarettes on the skin: he recommended psychiatric treatment, but the psychiatrist referred the patient back with the dry comment that a physical cause should be sought for a physical malady. Biopsy specimens were taken on three occasions: each time the histological picture was merely of a simple, unspecific, ulcerative inflammation. No organisms were seen either in the sections or in stained films of exudate from the ulcers. Swabs from the lesions were cultured on several occasions: various bacteria were grown, among them *Staphylococcus aureus, Proteus vulgaris* and *Pseudomonas pyocyanea,* but treatment with appropriate antibiotics was never of more than passing benefit. Two of the biopsy specimens were also cultured: both were reported as sterile, although the laboratory records when they were eventually reviewed were found to include a note that one of them had grown a 'peculiar yeast-like fungus, presumably a contaminant' that was not investigated further.

By the time when the patient met the pathologist at the party he had begun to regard the disease as beyond both diagnosis and cure. He readily enough accepted the pathologist's invitation to come to the lab. next day. There the clinical

picture was seen in all its classic simplicity, confirming the
diagnosis of ascending lymphangiitic sporotrichosis (Fig. 36.1)
that the pathologist had made to himself the evening before
from the characteristic history (see Chapter 37 for the cor-
ollary). It was a diagnosis he had been waiting nineteen years
to make, since being shown a case as a student in Ireland in
1935.[1]

A week later, the diagnosis had been confirmed by the
isolation of *Sporothrix schenckii* from an unulcerated nodule
freshly excised from the forearm. Three weeks later still,

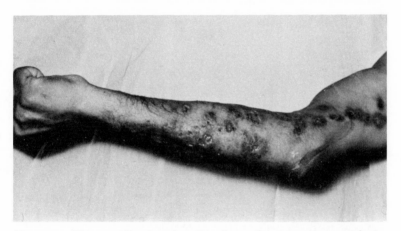

Fig. 36.1. The ascending lymphangiitic form of cutaneous sporotrichosis,
typical of the condition from which the law student suffered. The amateur
colour transparencies of the student's arm were badly lighted and are not fit to be
published: the illustration offered is of another case, but one that shows a clinical
condition that is practically identical.

The infection spreads in lymphatics from the site of inoculation. Focal granulomas develop in the subcutaneous tissue along their line: many become necrotic
and may then ulcerate, giving the picture shown. The lesion at the site of inoculation may persist, or may heal even while the granulomatous lymphangiitis
spreads.

Clinical photograph provided by Dr A. González Ochoa, Mexico City, and
reproduced by permission of Dr J. Edgar Morison, Editor of the *Ulster Medical
Journal* (the illustration was originally published in the article cited as Reference 1
on page 161).

From a 'Kodachrome' 35 mm transparency

after the patient had taken some 300 grams of sodium iodide by mouth (five grams three times a day), all the ulcers had become completely covered by epithelium and the inflammatory thickening of the tissues was appreciably less. Iodide was given for a further month in the same dose, and then withdrawn by progressively reducing the dose over another week.

There has been no recurrence of the disease since then (now twenty years past). There is unsightly scarring and pigmentation of the skin to mark where the lesions were, but no scarring or coloration of the patient's regard for the medical profession (which many of us have cause to be grateful for).

Sequels. In the reprehensible excitement of coming so unexpectedly on a case of sporotrichosis, the pathologist forgot his professional obligation to get in touch with the patient's own doctor before going any further. This earned him a chiding from his Dean, to whom the family doctor had complained, and an apology from the family doctor, who had not intended his pique to be taken too seriously (which it wasn't, in fact, which is worse).

The other sequel, rather later, was that the patient, so delighted to have the mystery of his disease solved and its manifestations so quickly overcome, sent a magnificent present to his hostess at the sherry party for her part in the history.

Comment

The mould that causes sporotrichosis, *Sporothrix schenckii,* is named for the Johns Hopkins medical student, Benjamin Robinson Schenck, who first recognized the infection, in 1896.* Its natural habitat is decaying vegetation, straw and

---

* It was another medical student, Alejandro Posadas, in Buenos Aires, who first recognized coccidioidomycosis, in 1891. Considering the small number of major deep-seated mycoses, medical students have done rather well to be responsible for the recognition of two so important as sporotrichosis and coccidioidomycosis.

soil, and, occasionally, living plants, including barbery, gorse and sphagnum moss. It enters the tissues through soiling of abrasions or the like, or when the skin is pierced by infected plant spines or thorns. The disease is either localized to the site of inoculation or, as in the law student's case, spreads along the regional lymphatics (though lymphadenitis is rarely a feature). Septicaemic and visceral infections are fortunately rare: their mortality is very high, whereas cutaneous sporotrichosis, though it may run a long course if untreated, seldom or never puts the patient's life in danger.

In sporotrichosis, unlike all the other deep fungal infections, the causative fungus can seldom be demonstrated in histological sections except by specific immunofluorescent staining, a procedure that is not generally available. Culture is therefore virtually the only straightforward means of confirming the diagnosis.

Footnote. Phaeosporotrichosis is a regrettable new name, used to refer to subcutaneous chromomycosis (chromomycotic 'cold abscess'). It means 'dark sporotrichosis', indicating that the causative organism, *Phialophora gougerotii*, is a brown fungus isolated from cases of subcutaneous infection that were regarded as a form of sporotrichosis: in fact, this condition has nothing to do with sporotrichosis.[2]

References

(1) Symmers, W. St C. (1968) Sporotrichosis in Ireland—a review. *Ulster Medical Journal, 37*, 85–101.
(2) Symmers, W. St C. (1971) New-style cold abscesses. *British Medical Journal, 2* (May 8), 337.

37 'También hay Jardines de Rosales en México'*

or The Great Occasion

> And my fause lover stole my rose,
> But ah! he left the thorn wi' me.
> (Burns, *Ye Banks and Braes o' Bonny Doon*)

The case of the young law student (page 156) had just been described in a talk on *Curiosa et Exotica* in Mexico City. The origin of the infection in a Dublin rose-garden prompted the chairman to interject what has therefore seemed an apt title for this chapter.

The Great Occasion of the subtitle was in England, not in Mexico, though it concerned a young Mexican doctor, who was for once himself the patient at a Grand Teaching Round in a small teaching hospital. However, it was not to the Mexican but to the pathologist that the occasion was great—the same pathologist who had met the law student at the sherry party in London. And the occasion was to be great to the pathologist because it gave him a chance to show off before his clinical colleagues and their students. And it gave him the chance to show off because he had heard the clinical history and seen the patient in advance, and he had confidently and dogmatically diagnosed to himself what was wrong and looked forward to the moment of triumph when he would

---

* There are also rose gardens in Mexico.

get up and in a few words solve his colleagues' diagnostic problem as if it were no problem at all.

The young Mexican's history and the clinical picture were those of a textbook case of the ascending lymphangiitic form of sporotrichosis. He had spent a holiday afternoon helping his mother to tend her rose garden at their home on the out-skirts of Mexico City. He had worked hard and happily, and his mother gave him as reward a bunch of fresh-cut roses to take to his future mother-in-law. Walking through the streets with the roses in his hand he met a group of his fellows out with their girls. They all went to a little café where there was a good deal of friendly banter between them. Later, when he got up to leave, one of the boys snatched at the bunch of roses, pulling it from his grasp so that a thorn tore deeply into the skin of the ball of one thumb. Soon, the bleed-ing stopped and the roses recovered, friendly abuse and greetings duly exchanged, the doctor went on his way.

Over the next few months he developed a series of chronic ulcers along the line of the subcutaneous lymphatics from the site of the scratch up to the middle of the inner aspect of the arm above the elbow. By this time he had arrived in England on an international bursary. The presence of the ulcers made clinical work inadvisable, so he consulted his obstetrical host who referred him to a surgical colleague who found the Wassermann to be negative and passed him on to a general physician who sought the opinion of the consultant dermatologist—who was abroad. The dermatological regi-strar thought inoculation tuberculosis the probable diagnosis but the laboratories could find no acid-fast bacilli and cultured only insignificant bacteria and a 'contaminant actinomyces' from the ulcers. Biopsy sections showed no evidence of tuberculosis, but just an unspecific chronic suppurative re-action—only H-and-E and ZN preparations were examined. So, the problem was put for diagnosis to the assembled talents of all who attended the Grand Teaching Round.

Came the afternoon of the Round and the Mexican presented his case history himself. The lesions were looked at by several of the doctors, one or two of whom were overheard in the safety of their places back among the audience to whisper certain grave diagnoses that they would not want to mention openly within earshot of the patient, particularly a patient who shared their professional knowledge. Most of the open discussion quickly focused on the 'contaminant actinomyces' and very soon actinomycosis was the general diagnostic consensus, in spite of the bacteriology registrar's objection that the patient's organism was aerobic and differed in other details from *Actinomyces israelii*.

Then the pathologist got up, suggested sporotrichosis, supported this with photographs of proved cases, referred to the frequency of the disease in Mexico and generally tied all the observations in with this diagnosis. The response of his colleagues was generous and heart-warming. Even the sceptical scientists among them seemed impressed, once the patient had explained that he knew nothing of sporotrichosis himself, because he had not studied medicine in his own country but in a school in a part of the United States where this mycosis would be about as infrequent in clinical practice as it is in Britain.

Humble Pie. The actinomycete turned out to be *Nocardia brasiliensis,* not a contaminant but the cause of the young Mexican's disease, which was not sporotrichosis but a rather unusual lymphangiitic form of nocardial mycetoma (see page 154). The infection gradually responded to treatment with long-acting sulphonamides, and all that now remains is the pigmented scarring where the ulcers were.

Comment

Like *Sporothrix schenckii* (see page 160), *Nocardia brasiliensis* may enter the tissues on infected thorns and the like. The colonies of the organism, which are usually small, are quite readily found in sections of the lesions. Review of the biopsy in the Mexican doctor's case showed them immediately in Gram-stained sections but without difficulty in the HE ones too. The pathologist's prime mistake was that he didn't keep quiet until he had had a chance to look at the biopsy sections for himself—he still flushes at the memory of his first glance at the HE section, for the first field (as luck so often has it) had an unmistakable colony of *Nocardia brasiliensis* at its centre (Fig. 37.1).

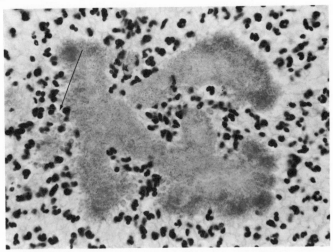

Fig. 37.1.   A colony of *Nocardia brasiliensis* in an abscess in the biopsy specimen. This photograph shows the deflationary centre of the first field that the pathologist looked at with the microscope, having already foolishly committed himself to a diagnosis of sporotrichosis on clinical grounds (he wasn't even a clinical pathologist). The identity of the colony, never histologically in doubt, was confirmed by isolating the organism in cultures.

The colony shown here, characteristically slightly denser at its periphery, has a fine punctate structure because the nocardia is present mainly as short bacillary filaments. At some points at the surface of the colony there are homogeneous eosinophile 'clubs' (arrow): these are of the same nature as the corresponding structures in colonies of *Actinomyces israelii* (Fig. 1.3, page 3) and of actinobacilli (Fig. 1.1, facing page 2) and those that participate in the formation of candida asteroids and comparable bodies (Fig. 2.2, page 8).

Haematoxylin–eosin   × 475

Memorandum. This type of *Nocardia brasiliensis* infection *must* be remembered in the differential diagnosis of lymphangiitic sporotrichosis. *Ipse dixit*.

38 Erinaceus and the Sandal

Sandals are usually light and cool, often cheap, and sometimes very comfortable. Worn on appropriate occasions, especially over socks or stockings, they need not be unaesthetic, except through vulgarity of design, materials or colour. Only the particular can wear them inoffensively on otherwise bare feet, and even they will find the dust of the road soon tediously evident.

Sandals protect the feet better than no footwear at all. But they have been known to fail to divert leeches and scorpions and ants, snakes and hookworm larvae, broken glass and tetanus spores and thorn-borne fungi, and sea-urchin spines and the spines of that other urchin, *Erinaceus* the hedgehog. This is the story of the erinaceous encounter—it happened in England, not Ireland.

A young woman, barefoot but for open-toed sandals, was walking quickly along a poorly lit surburban road in Warwickshire one night when she stumbled over a hedgehog that she saw, just too late to avoid it, curled up in her path. She felt immediate pain in the middle toe of the foot that struck the animal. When she got home, a few minutes later, she saw what looked like a splinter under the toenail, broken off at the free edge of the nail and reaching almost to its root. Domestically available tools proving too coarse, she went at once to her doctor, who had no difficulty in pulling out what proved to be one of the hedgehog's spines.

Within a few days an abscess had formed under the nail. The doctor's attempts to establish drainage by cutting away a narrow wedge of nail along the festering track failed. A course of penicillin had no effect. Nine days after the injury the nail was avulsed under general anaesthesia. The nailbed did not heal: within three weeks there was a granulating ulcer involving the whole of the distal two thirds of the dorsum of the toe. Thin seropurulent discharge seeped from the raw surface and the tissues were swollen and indurated. The patient found the condition more incommoding than painful; her general health was unaffected.

Cultures of exudate from the ulcer grew a few colonies of a penicillin-sensitive strain of coagulase-producing *Staphylococcus aureus,* but nothing else. A second course of penicillin had no effect. Seven weeks after the encounter with the hedgehog a slightly tender nodule formed under the skin just proximal to the base of the affected toe; the area round it became puffy and red. For the first time, sporotrichosis was thought of: and *Sporothrix schenckii* was cultured from the drop of matter that was aspirated from the nodule.

Large doses of potassium iodide were given by mouth. Within three weeks the ulcerated surface was completely covered by epithelium and the nodule had disappeared. To prevent recurrence of the infection the treatment was continued for twelve weeks. That was twelve years ago: there has been no trouble since. The toenail did not regenerate, but thanks to the standard products of the cosmetics industry only the patient and her doctors know the truth when she wears toeless sandals, which, it is reported, she still does.

Comment

Presumably the fungus was carried by the hedgehog on its skin, picked up perhaps from earth or infected plants. As sporotrichosis, like mycetoma (see page 139, footnote), can be acquired through pricks by contaminated thorns, the circumstances of this patient's inoculation, piquant as they were, are but a variation on a familiar theme (see page 161).

For the record, sporotrichosis has not yet been recognized in a hedgehog. And no one has considered in depth the role of the pocket torch in the prophylaxis of disease.

39 The Pluffer[1]

A schoolboy in Belfast, in 1929, was hit in one eye by a pellet of sago or the like, projected from a pluffer.* The injury caused a small bruise over the sclera, a few millimetres lateral to the limbus. Generalized conjunctivitis developed during the following week, accompanied by much hyperaemia and oedema. The site of impact became superficially ulcerated. The family doctor advised frequent bathing of the eye with a boric acid lotion and the instillation of drops of silver nitrate solution. By a fortnight after the injury most of the conjunctival reaction had subsided but the 'ulster' had enlarged to about five millimetres in diameter and there was marked dilatation of the blood vessels round the cornea. The child complained increasingly of pain in the eye and of blurring of sight.

He was not seen by an oculist until four weeks after the injury. By then there was severe iridocyclitis, a hypopyon and

---

* The 'pluffer' was standard pocket armament among otherwise reasonably responsible children in some schools in Belfast, and doubtless elsewhere in the world, possibly under other names, at the end of the 1920s. For all I know, it still may be so. It was a straight piece of laboratory glass tubing, five to ten centimetres long and of a bore appropriate for the average grain of sago, barley or rice, the usual ammunition (Fig. 39.1). The propellant was air, forcibly expelled from the mouth into the loaded breech of the weapon, which was held in the lips and aimed in the general direction of blackboard, windows, lamps or schoolfellows (rarely, masters).

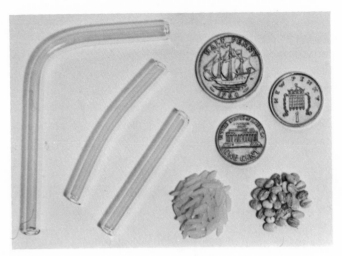

Fig. 39.1. Three pluffers, and ammunition (barley and rice). Two pennies and a make, for size.

Mise en scène *and photography by Mr R. S. Barnett*

corneal clouding. The disease worsened. After another two weeks the eye was removed: there was no possibility of its sight recovering, and there was the risk of sympathetic ophthalmia.

Cultures from the interior of the eye gave a pure growth of *Sporothrix schenckii.* The histological picture—suppurative and tuberculoid granulomatous tissue—was that of sporotrichosis: as usual in this infection, no organisms were seen in the sections.

The postoperative course was uncomplicated. There was no residual infection in the orbit. The feared possibility of sympathetic ophthalmia did not materialize.

Later, back at school, the boy shockingly fascinated his schoolmates by taking out his artificial eye at thruppence, or two one-D nuggets,* a look.

* Nuggett: a chocolate-covered bar of nougat, costing a penny (1/240th of £1) in the tuckshop.

Sequel. In 1940 the patient volunteered for the RAF and somehow managed to be passed fit for flying duties. He became a navigator, and continued to hide his disability successfully. He was several times decorated for gallantry before being posted missing on a reconnaissance flight.

Comment

Ocular sporotrichosis is very rare, though frequent enough to deserve particular notice among the mycotic diseases of the eyes. However, it is far from the most important ocular mycosis, this position belonging to the various forms of keratomycosis, the primary infections of the cornea by species of *Aspergillus, Curvularia, Cephalosporium* and other fungi. In common with these infections the prognosis is reasonably good, provided the infection is recognized early enough and then appropriately treated: otherwise, at best sight is endangered and too often blindness results, from corneal opacity or from penetration of the bulb.

The source of the boy's infection is uncertain. The missile that struck his eye may have carried the fungus, or the infection may have been caused subsequently by invasion of the injured tissue. The fungal flora of samples of sago, rice and barley carried by his schoolmates, and by him, as ammunition for pluffers included several moulds, but no potential pathogens. He had none of the interests that might have carried a special risk of exposure to infection from soil or plants and other vegetable matter, the usual habitats of *Sporothrix schenckii*. He lived in a gardenless part of the city, seldom went to the parks or country and avoided outdoor games. All in all, it is likeliest that the shot from the pluffer was the means of infection.

References

(1) Craig, J. A., Houston, T. Symmers [Belfast], W. St C. (1968) Contemporaneous notes on this case, cited as Case 4 in Symmers, W. St C. (1968) Sporotrichosis in Ireland—a review. *Ulster Medical Journal, 37*, 85–101.
(2) Gordon, D. M. (1947) Ocular sporotrichosis—report of a case. *Archives of Ophthalmology, 37* (January), 56–72.

40 The Part Greater than the Whole[1]

The patient whose case this chapter records lived, like the boy in Chapter 39, in Northern Ireland. Like him, she died on active service. She was a woman of means: at the start of this history she was living as a recluse, though in substantial comfort. When she went out, which was rarely, she dressed in a long-outdated fashion with voluminous skirts and a flaring coat. She was regarded in the neighbourhood as a little touched.

One day she sent for a doctor. He had not met her before. She told him her time had come. He mistook her meaning, and remarked that she looked as one who had many years' enjoyment of life to look forward to. Gently, she corrected his misunderstanding: she had meant, she said, that she was in labour—though an old maid, she had been pregnant for many years, she said, and now the time of her confinement was come. The doctor demurred, kindly, assuming her to be a little odd in her mind; impatient now, she demanded that he examine her to learn for himself that what she said was correct.

Her abdomen was greatly distended and tense, contrasting with the emaciation of her chest and limbs. The veins beneath the skin of her trunk were uncommonly conspicuous, and there was a fine net of small vessels over the costal margins. The doctor's first impression was that his new patient must have cirrhosis with gross ascites. She refused to let him send her to hospital, resentful of his inability to appreciate the reality of what she had told him.

Gradually, over the following days, the doctor got her trust. She told him the history of her 'pregnancy'. Her abdomen had started to swell some fifteen years before, when she was approaching 50. At the time she was fashion director of a Mayfair company. Her work often took her to Paris, where she had an apartment. When the enlargement of her abdomen became noticeable her associates all too readily deduced a scandal. Soon an influential small section of her clientèle began to take their custom to rival houses. She had to resign, or—as she put it to the doctor—for the baby's sake she had to give up working. In the seclusion of her retirement she accepted her pregnancy as a miraculous favour of St Joan, whose land for a while had been her second home.

At last the doctor persuaded her to go into hospital. But soon after her admission a manic state developed, precipitated by the realization that she was in a general ward and not in the maternity department. This extra strain on her frail physical condition nearly killed her, but with devoted nursing she pulled through. By this time it had been recognized that her abdominal distension was not ascitic but due to some multilocular cystic mass, probably an ovarian tumour. Once she was thought strong enough, this diagnosis was confirmed at laparotomy: the stomach and bowel and the solid organs were spread thinly over the tense surface of an immense tumour arising from one ovary. The tumour was removed in one piece, the operation eased by aspirating the contents of some of the cystic compartments. The patient was seriously shocked after the operation, but recovered.

Histological examination showed that the tumour was a

benign mucinous cystadenoma. Its weight on removal from the patient was thirty-five kilograms (and that was after aspiration of the contents of some of its locules). On the day before the operation the patient had weighed sixty-seven kilograms; seven days after it she weighed twenty-nine kilograms and six months later fifty-nine kilograms.

She was transformed both physically and mentally by the operation. Her convalescence and rehabilitation were completed by spending some months in France. She then returned to the North of Ireland and began to take an active part in voluntary welfare work there. Soon she was to accept the challenge of taking part in the organization of air-raid relief. When the war eventually came she was transferred at her own request to one of the more vulnerable urban areas in England. Her name had appeared in more than one Honours List before she was killed while driving an ambulance during a bombardment.

Reference

(1) Kirk, T. S. (1935) An unpublished case, quoted in *Systemic Pathology*, 1st edition (1966), edited by G. Payling Wright and W. St C. Symmers, volume 1, page 852. London: Longmans.

41 The Invisible Giant . . .

A girl of 18 came to hospital to start her training as a nurse. At her first health check the staff doctor was surprised when examining her heart to find a large, firm mass in her left breast. She was otherwise well, although much overweight. Her bust was large, and in spite of the tumour on the left there was no asymmetry. She seemed not to have been aware of any anomaly.

The surgeon who was asked to see her recognized the tumour to be a 'giant fibroadenoma'. He removed it through a short incision below the breast. Immediately after the operation there was marked asymmetry, due to the loss of bulk from the breast that had been operated on. The tumour was a rather flattened sphere, its longest dimension nine centimetres (Fig. 41.1); it weighed just under 550 grams.

When she came back to hospital after her sick-leave, five weeks after the operation, her breasts were again symmetrical. Presumably, fatty tissue had proliferated to fill the space left by removal of the tumour.

Side Effect. Like most doctors and nurses (and others?) who become patients in hospital, she was understandably inquisitive about her case notes, and at last she got an opportunity to read them. By ill luck, the pathologist who had dealt with her specimen was of an older school and had used the expression 'cystosarcoma phyllodes' in his histological description of what in fact he recognized to be a benign

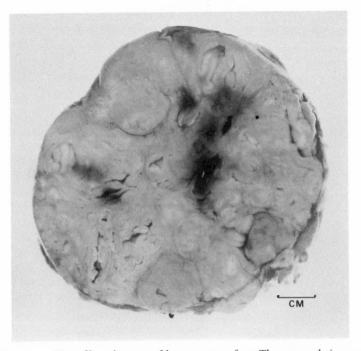

Fig. 41.1.   Giant fibroadenoma of breast, cut surface. The encapsulation and nodular structure are seen, with compressed spaces lined by epithelium and the characteristic gyrate appearance resulting from disproportionate growth of the connective tissue components. The areas of haemorrhage are artefacts, occurring during the surgical manipulation of the tumour.

growth (Fig. 41.2).* The patient was already familiar enough with the medical vocabulary to know that 'sarcoma' is used of a form of cancer. What she did not know, then, was that the word, coined long before the microscopical structure of tissues was discovered, had originally described any fleshy mass, not necessarily cancerous, and that it persists in that sense in a few historic names for particular tumours that in

---

* Giant fibroadenoma of breast has several other synonyms, some of them every bit as objectionable as cystosarcoma. Cystadenosarcoma, adenofibrosarcoma, giant intra-canalicular myxoma and Brodie's serocystic disease are among the terms that still have some currency.

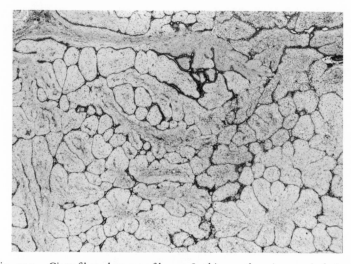

Fig. 41.2.   Giant fibroadenoma of breast. In this case the microscopical picture was everywhere typical of the intracanalicular variety of the common mammary fibroadenoma, only the overall size of the tumour distinguishing it from one of these. The dark network represents the two facing layers of epithelium compressed together by the connective tissue masses that they cover. In contrast to the usual finding in giant fibroadenomas, the connective tissue component is more fibrotic than cellular (though more cellular than in the average conventional fibroadenoma).

Haematoxylin–eosin   × 20

fact are generally benign. It was some time before she was relieved of the distress that looking through her notes had caused. Her fright was needless, for her tumour was altogether benign in structure.

Outcome. It is nineteen years since this episode. She has had no more trouble. She completed her training, losing most of her surplus weight in doing so. She married and has reared a family. There were no feeding problems, on either side.

Comments

The giant fibroadenoma of breast is a rare tumour, in contrast to the commonplace fibroadenomas that every medical student so soon becomes familiar with. Its relation to the small tumours is obscure. In a minority of cases, perhaps up to ten per cent, giant fibroadenoma behaves as a cancer, metastasizing. It is seldom possible to forecast which tumours will do so, for most giant fibroadenomas are very cellular and many are also cytologically pleomorphic, in spite of the usually good prognosis. It is only a few that are so fully differentiated that one can confidently recognize them as benign. The nurse's tumour was one of these.

Hers was a comparatively small giant. The largest that I have seen was twenty-five centimetres in its longest dimension and weighed just on five kilograms. The next chapter is concerned with the other extreme.

42 . . . and the Troublesome Dwarf

An intelligent middle-aged woman, active in her profession, had lived for some years in the USA. There she had acquired a degree of health-consciousness that is still rare in any group of lay people in Britain. She attended an executives' health centre every three months for an exhaustive clinical, cardiographic, radiological, biochemical and cytological overhaul. She had also been schooled in various procedures for self-examination. These included regular use of Albustix, Azostix, Clinitest, Hemastix, Ictotest and Occultest, as well as palpating her breasts every few days in accordance with an almost ritual pattern.

One day she discovered a small nodule at the periphery of one breast. She went to her doctor at once. At first he had difficulty in finding the nodule, but with her help he eventually felt it as an indistinct small body, at most a couple of millimetres across, that rolled under the finger tip like a tiny piece of shot between skin and chest wall. At the patient's insistence it was excised. The sections showed it to be a minute fibroadenoma-like focus (Fig. 42.1).

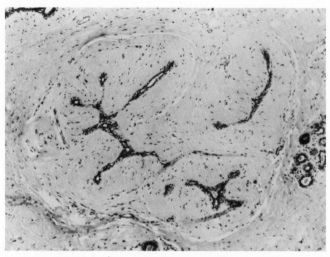

Fig. 42.1. This is the tiny fibroadenoma-like focus that caused the patient so much worry—a millimetre and a quarter by a millimetre in its longest dimensions. Its structure is that of an intracanalicular fibroadenoma, but it is not a tumour. Small foci like this are far from rare as one of several patterns of disturbance of the balance between epithelial and stromal tissue in breasts pathologically affected by cyclical or other functional influences. What is exceptional is that a lesion so minute should attract attention. See Figs 13.1 and 13.2. also (pages 48 and 49).

Haematoxylin–eosin   × 65.

Months passed before the patient conceded that the doctors had not been keeping the truth from her and that the nodule was indeed benign. Since then she has had several more 'scares' through discovering nodules in various parts of both breasts. Luckily, her doctors have succeeded in teaching her that such findings, while never to be treated with contempt, are common and need commonsense attention, and that surgery is not automatically made necessary by the finding of a 'lump'.

Coincidence. It is salutary to learn that this woman developed diabetes. This was diagnosed only after her admission to a hospital in coma. Once she was well enough to review what had happened, it turned out that she had switched from Clinitest to Clinistix and had been confused about the significance of the colour changes when using the latter—she had thought it normal for the test area of the strip to be coloured blue after its dip in urine, having been accustomed to the blue of Clinitest normality.

43 The Reciprocating Dermoid[1]

A woman of 40 noticed a lump in her neck. It grew slowly and after six months was excised for diagnosis. It was a secondary deposit of well-differentiated papillary thyroid carcinoma. A week later the surgeon, assuming that the primary tumour would be in the corresponding lateral lobe of the thyroid, as is usual in such cases, operated to remove the lobe and isthmus. While freeing the isthmus, which in this case was a well-defined bridge of glandular tissue linking the lateral lobes, he found a discrete nodule, about half a centimetre in diameter, in the line of his dissection. An immediate frozen section confirmed his suspicion that this was a primary thyroid carcinoma. As careful slicing of the excised lateral lobe showed no macroscopical tumour the surgeon concluded that the isthmic focus must be the source of the metastasis: in view of its median situation and the possibility of spread to the other side of the neck as well, he decided to make the thyroidectomy total, removing the other lateral lobe. The lymph nodes were dissected from both sides of the neck at the same time. Sections showed no tumour in the nodes or in the lateral lobes of the thyroid. No other treatment was given.

The patient was put on thyroid extract at a daily dose of 120 milligrams. She kept so well that she found it difficult to believe that the tablets were necessary. However, she took them unfailingly until two years after the operation. At that time she had to cope with an emotional crisis that was probably not related to her health: as a result she settled abroad, where she became involved with a religious group opposed to medical methods of treatment. Under this influence she stopped taking the thyroid extract—she kept perfectly well. A year or so later she became critical of the teachings of her new acquaintances and broke with their church. As she felt so fit she saw no point in resuming the treatment.

Her health continued to be seemingly good for the next five years, apart from the onset of metrorrhagia toward the end of that time. The bleeding was due to endometrial hyperplasia associated with follicular ovarian cysts: the uterus, tubes and ovaries were removed. She was then 48; it was eight years since the thyroidectomy. A characteristic dermoid cyst, six centimetres across, was an incidental finding in one ovary: most of its solid parts consisted of mature thyroid tissue, indistinguishable from the normal gland. A year later she was in a piteous state from myxoedema. At first the manifestations of hypothyroidism were attributed to the surgical menopause, but giving oestrogen did not affect them. Then, one day, her doctor noticed for the first time the almost invisible surgical scar on her neck and realized its significance (and also that once again he, like many another of us, had overlooked the quite typical if not yet full-blown picture of myxoedema).

Substitution therapy with thyroxine was carefully worked up to a daily dose of 0·3 milligrams. This fully restored her health. She remains well—and very conscientious about taking her tablets.

Comment

Instances of a tumour functioning to the benefit of its host are rare. In this case the tumour was a teratoma, an ovarian 'dermoid', which some would not regard as a neoplasm at all. It is therefore worth recalling that in exceptional circumstances even cancerous deposits have acted comparably. In a classic, though unpublished, case in the decade of the First World War, the secretion of a very slowly growing secondary tumour in the sacrum enabled a patient to continue in public life for several years after total removal of the thyroid for cancer. The patient had been dilatory about taking the prescribed thyroid extract and eventually stopped doing so, with such lack of the threatened consequences that the doctors were accused publicly of fraudulent prescribing—it was a celebrated suit, and possibly symptomatic. Sepsis after ulceration of the metastasis was the eventual cause of death.

Reference

(1) Hughesdon, P. E. & Symmers, W. St C. (1968) In *Systemic Pathology*, 1st edition, edited by G. Payling Wright and W. St C. Symmers, page 856. London: Longmans.

44 Cardiac Catheterization

A young mother was admitted to the medical wards of a general hospital for investigation of symptoms that her family doctor had diagnosed as due to a gastric ulcer. The ward to which she was admitted was, at the time, engaged in an investigation designed to establish the range of normal findings on cardiac catheterization: for this purpose every second patient admitted with other than a cardiovascular or respiratory disease was included in the study (the numbers were arbitrarily limited in this way because the facilities available did not allow of including every such patient).

Permission to carry out the investigation was not specifically asked of the patients. This was thought unnecessary by the investigators in view of the hospital's rule that every patient on admission was obliged to sign, or in lieu of signature to append a mark to, a 'Statement of Obligation'. This statement gave prominence to its requirement for such personal data as the patient's full name, sex, age, address and religion, the name, address and occupation of the nearest of kin and the address of the police or coast guard station nearest to the nearest of kin's home if there was no means of telephonic communication directly to the latter. In smaller print were regulations about visiting hours, non-admittance of pets and children as visitors, procedure for handing in flowers and other permitted gifts for patients, and a list of prohibited gifts (including medicines, contraceptives, political and religious pamphlets and pictures other than religious pamphlets and pictures the gift of recognized religious officers, and 'spirituous liquors as Geneva and strong ale').

Also among the abundant small print on this two-page document, and without preamble or separate heading, sandwiched in one paragraph between notes on borrowing books from the mobile hospital library and on the need to give notice before admission of special diets for 'those sick of particular religious persuasions', was the advice: 'When appropriate sectio cadaveris will be carried out unless the nearest of kin shall have given contrary notice not less than 24 hours before exitus (up to 72 hours the week-end intervening) that he or she decline this service provided without charge at the hospital's discretion'.

Elsewhere, again in the small print of the 'Statement of Obligation', was a further warning to those able to read and understand it as such: 'All investigations and treatments considered desirable by the visiting doctors and their delegate representatives shall be accepted by the patient and refusal thereof shall discharge the hospital and the doctors from all responsibility to the patient who by such refusal shall be deemed to have discharged his or her self from further sojourn in and attendance on the hospital's practice.'

And much else besides contributed to the length of a document that, very properly, has ceased to be used.

The patient whose story is this chapter's theme turned out to have a chronic gastric ulcer. She was also one of the 'every second patient' group and so cardiac catheterization was performed. Once the various measurements and samples had been taken the physician started to withdraw the catheter: almost at once he felt resistance to his pull upon it, and try as he would, though gently, he could not make it come. He repeated his careful pull once he had the catheter under observation on the X-ray screen—its tip was seen still to be within the heart, lodged at a point corresponding to the tricuspid valve and showing only such excursion as the natural movements of the valve might cause.

The physician asked his chief's advice, and the chief called in the thoracic surgeon. The surgeon tugged very gently on the catheter and it suddenly came free: he continued to pull on it until it stuck again, this time in the vein through which it had been introduced. He cut down and opened the vein: the catheter came out, its tip looped into a simple knot.

Penicillin had already established its place in the treatment of bacterial endocarditis. The patient was therefore given a good course of the drug, a precaution in case the catheter had damaged the tricuspid valve, for it seemed likely that the knot had caught in the chordae tendineae. She never showed any evidence of damage to the heart or of infection. I never heard the outcome of her gastric ulceration.

In the circumstances, the misadventure with the catheter was thought not to be of enough scientific interest to warrant publication.

Comment

I am told that it is impossible for a cardiac catheter to become knotted.

Mutatis mutandis . . . The doctors concerned with another patient's cardiac catheterization ruled that the procedure had had nothing to do with an illness that began almost three months afterwards with symptoms that eventually proved to be due to candida endocarditis of the tricuspid valve. In the circumstances, her case was thought not to warrant publication either. She died after an illness lasting nine weeks. Her catheterization had been part of a fact-finding investigation similar to the one already mentioned. She and her family did not know what the procedure was: they took it to be a 'blood test', part of the investigation of the minor psychiatric illness that was the reason for her being in hospital. Her GP was not told about it as it was not relevant to the illness that had caused him to send her to hospital. That he did not know of the catheterization possibly contributed to the delay in recognition of the endocarditis.

The diagnosis was delayed further because after her readmission to the hospital a classic error in laboratory interpretation occurred—when the blood cultures repeatedly gave a pure growth of a candida this result was repeatedly misattributed to air-borne contamination. But those were days when candida septicaemia was not widely known, and when candida endocarditis was beyond hope of effective treatment . . .

45 Cotton Embolism

A man of about 30 had recurrent symptoms suggesting chronic pyelonephritis. Intravenous pyelography showed no definite abnormality except for moderate dilatation of the lowermost calices of the left renal pelvis. It was thought that renal arteriography might be more helpful: the first attempt failed because of obstruction to the flow of the radio-opaque medium (sodium acetrizoate) through the catheter—in her anxiety to make the injection in the three to four seconds that should not be exceeded if the technique is to be successful, the radiologist pumped quite strongly against the resistance that she felt, thus clearing the obstruction, but too late for good pictures to be obtained as the earlier fraction of the dose had already been excreted.

The investigation was successful at the second attempt, some days later. An unusual distribution of vessels about the lower pole of the left kidney was shown. There was also an apparently complete blockage of an artery in the lower pole of the right kidney. It was decided to have a surgical look at the kidneys in order to determine whether the abnormal parts should be removed.

For family reasons it was two months before the patient could return to hospital for the operation. An accessory renal artery was found on the left side, apparently rising from a lumbar artery. The aberrant vessel compressed the necks of the lower calices, which were thickened and dilated; there

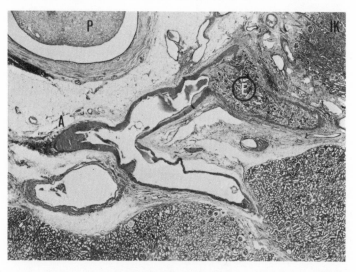

Fig. 45.1.   Section across the renal sinus in the resected part of the left kidney. The bifurcation of a lobar artery is marked (A). The upper interlobar branch of this vessel is completely obstructed at its bifurcation by an organizing granuloma, the reaction to the cotton wool embolus (E). The granuloma is seen to fill the lower branch of the affected artery: the other branch is not in the plane of the section.

The parenchyma in the upper right corner of the field (IK) is in part infarcted and atrophic. There are no significant abnormalities of the region supplied by the unoccluded branch of the lobar artery (across the bottom of the field).

P, a normal papilla within a calyx.

See Figs 45.2 to 45.4.

Haematoxylin–eosin   ×9

was considerable scarring of the lower pole of the kidney but no abnormality elsewhere. On the right side there were no obvious anomalies of the renal vessels, but in the lower pole of the kidney there was a large, hyperaemic, triangular depression, evidently a scar developing after an infarct. The lower pole of each kidney was removed.

The piece of the left kidney showed chronic pyelonephritis, presumably from infection complicating obstruction of the calices by the accessory artery.

The lesion in the lower pole of the right kidney was an organizing infarct, the result of plugging of a branch of the renal artery by an embolus of cotton (Figs 45.1 to 45.4). It seems likely that a piece of cotton wool, perhaps used in

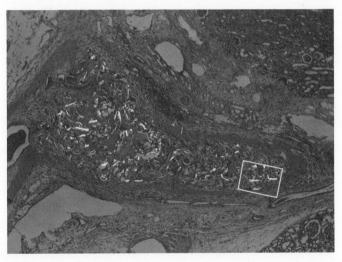

Fig. 45.2. The occluded part of the artery in Fig. 45.1 has been photographed at a higher magnification in polarized light. The analysing filter was rotated short of complete extinction so that sufficient detail of the tissue can be seen to enable the landmarks to be recognized. The bright material in the granuloma is cotton, part of the cotton wool embolus (see text).

The field within the marked rectangle is shown at higher magnification in Figs 45.3 and 45.4.

Haematoxylin–eosin × 20

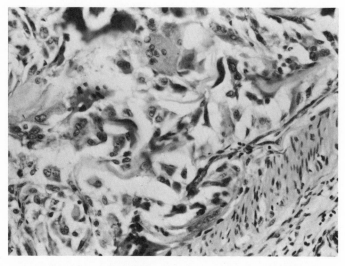

Fig. 45.3.   This is the rectangular area marked in Fig. 45.2, magnified nine times. The muscle of the wall of the occluded artery crosses the lower right corner of the field. The organizing granuloma in the lumen is formed of mononucleate and multinucleate macrophages. The cotton fibres can be identified by comparing this picture with Fig. 45.4, which shows the same field in polarized light.

Haematoxylin–eosin   × 180

cleaning the arteriography set, had been forced into the lumen of the catheter in such a way that the obstruction was not noticed until after starting to inject the medium at the first attempt to carry out the arteriography. Dislodged by the radiologist's misguided efforts to clear the obstruction, its passage into the renal artery would explain the subsequent findings.

The patient has been free from symptoms since his operation, now eight years ago.

Comment

This is one of two practically identical cases of renal embolism by cotton wool that I have seen in different hospitals. Renal

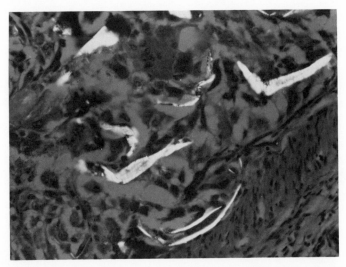

Fig. 45.4. The field of Fig. 45.3, photographed in polarized light through an analyser rotated short of complete extinction. The doubly refractile fragments of cotton fibre are shown clearly (compare with Fig. 45.2 also).

Haematoxylin–eosin × 180

arteriography seems to have been the origin of the embolus in both cases.

Memorabilium. In older days, it was not unusual to give an intravenous infusion of glucose saline, or even blood, simply by pouring the fluid into an open-topped cylindrical glass funnel connected through rubber tubing to a needle in a vein. In following this procedure it was sometimes the practice to filter the saline or blood by pouring it through sterile cotton gauze covering the mouth of the funnel. Sometimes the neck of the funnel was designed to hold a small plug of cotton wool or gauze as an extra filter. Not surprisingly, minute granulomas could sometimes be found when the lungs were carefully searched histologically after such methods of infusion had been used. The granulomas were not numerous enough to hinder the circulation or large enough to cause significant scarring; the pathologists who recognized their occurrence did not consider them of practical importance. Obviously, the pulmonary lesions caused by such minute pieces of cotton washed off the filters are not comparable with the infarcts caused by the much larger emboli accompanying renal arteriography in the two cases referred to here.

46 Sternal Puncture

An elderly woman, suspected of having a megaloblastic anaemia, was to have a sternal marrow examination. The trainee pathologist whose job it was to obtain the specimen had already done some dozens of sternal punctures and had been well schooled in the procedure, its possible hazards and the precautions to take. Yet, in spite of his care, this patient's sternum snapped across, a couple of centimetres below the point in the manubrium where he had started to press the needle home.

The patient was immediately distressed by the fright and the pain. She was given a small dose of morphine. A watch was kept on her heart rate, jugular venous pressure and systemic arterial pressure. As feared, evidence of cardiac tamponade began to show. The cardiologist and the thoracic surgeon had been called, and everything was ready for a surgical exploration of the pericardial sac under conditions as good as could have been hoped for in emergency.

When the pericardium was opened, part of its parietal layer was found to have been nipped between the broken ends of the sternum. There was brisk oozing of blood from the crushed and partly torn tissue—about eighty millilitres of blood and blood clot were removed from the sac. The damaged pericardial tissue was excised. No attempt was made to fix the fracture surgically as the apposed ends seemed in firm contact.

The patient's recovery was uninterrupted. The diagnosis of pernicious anaemia was confirmed (marrow from an iliac crest helped in this) and the response to treatment was predictably excellent.

47 Cisternal Puncture

A young physician was asked by a group of junior colleagues whom he was coaching for Membership if he would demonstrate cisternal puncture. He had been well trained in this procedure himself by a carefully dexterous neurologist, and he had performed it many times without mishap. As there were several patients in the ward whose cerebrospinal fluid had to be examined he agreed to the request.

He tapped two patients' cisterns easily, explaining every detail of what he was doing. Then, rashly, he asked if any one in the group would like to try the technique. He regretted this impulsive offer at once, but felt he could not go back on it, for already the most pushing man among them was scrubbing up. While waiting for the next patient to be brought to the operating room, the instructor went through the steps of the tap again, at each point mentioning the possible snags and dangers, particularly the risk of the needle going too deep.

'Right', he said to his pupil, when all was ready, 'Now, you're quite clear what you have to do? OK—go ahead.' The younger doctor lifted the needle, aligned it accurately, and thrust it quickly through the anaesthetized area of skin, through the subcutaneous tissue and the ligaments, through the 'brown paper' resistance of the dura mater, across the great cistern and—within a second of piercing the skin—deep into the medulla oblongata. The patient died instantly.

48 Lumbar Puncture

A young woman with multiple sclerosis was in hospital for the first time. Her illness had been diagnosed on unarguable clinical grounds, and as the history and findings were characteristic she was invited to spend a few days as an in-patient so that she might be used as a 'clinical case' in a prize examination for senior medical students. The teachers organizing the exam. thought it essential for this purpose to have the results of certain laboratory and other studies available in case any candidate asked for them, even though the physician who had looked after the patient had not felt any need for them in practice. Among these was a lumbar puncture, which showed no abnormality.

Acute suppurative meningitis followed the lumbar puncture, due to infection by *Staphylococcus albus,** an organism ordinarily found among the flora of the skin and generally to be regarded as non-pathogenic. The leptomeninges are notoriously vulnerable to infection introduced directly from outside, even when the organisms concerned have little or no pathogenicity under other circumstances: this is probably

---

* For the record, this strain was a non-chromogenic, non-haemolytic, coagulase-negative, gelatinase-negative staphylococcus that produced only trivial local lesions on inoculation into laboratory animals.

because the 'blood–brain barrier' hinders access of antibodies and other protective substances.

It is likely that this woman's infection resulted from a failure in aseptic technique when the lumbar puncture was done.

The response to treatment was slow, although the staphylococcus was sensitive to penicillin and appropriate doses were given intramuscularly and intrathecally. The symptoms of multiple sclerosis rapidly became severer at this time. Interference with bladder control was followed by cystitis and pyelonephritis from *Escherichia coli* infection. The patient died of these complications some weeks after recovery from the meningitis.

Footnote. Qualifying and postgraduate clinical examinations to test the knowledge and competence of candidates for degrees and diplomas are nowadays conducted with every regard for the safety, comfort and sensibilities of the patients —and doubtless they almost always have been. In the past, it has been known for patients to suffer unnecessarily at the hands of candidates, either through the unwonted nervousness of the latter or because of maladroit and unsupervised physical examination. Among such events recalled from personal knowledge, though by good fortune not from personal participation, are: fatal heart failure from laying an orthopnoeic patient flat; fatal heart failure from sitting a patient upright so that a ball thrombus impacted in the mitral orifice (it could have happened at any time); fatal hyperthyroid crisis (from over-palpation of a toxic goitre); pulmonary embolism (not fatal) while feeling the calves for evidence of deep vein thrombosis: fracture of ribs (from over-vigorous examination of an old man's chest); rupture of a malarial spleen (from over-anxious prodding for its edge under the costal margin when it was a hand's breadth nearer the umbilicus); rupture of the fetal membranes in late pregnancy (from excessively hard palpation of the uterus);

and ante-partum placental separation (while trying too desperately to decide the fetal lie.).

49 *Duodenal Aspiration*

A great surgeon was commonly regarded as a cold and crusty character. Behind this reputation was a sensitive and gentle man, his real nature evident to his patients more than to most of his colleagues. One day he found himself faced with the unavoidable prospect of doing a cystoscopy when his usual anaesthetist was unrecallably on holiday (unjustifiably, but understandably, the surgeon trusted no one else to anaesthetize his patients). Only an inadvertence could have explained the anaesthetist's absence while the surgeon was still about: the inadvertence was that the latter had forgotten, inconceivably, the long-arranged follow-up appointment with a papillec-tomized patient. The patient was an opinionated and bully-ing member of the hospital's 'Penny Council',* a body since defunct but in those days powerful in its corporate capacity to control, coercively rather than constitutionally, some of the affairs of an institution dependent entirely on voluntary contributions. It was typical of the patient that he had bridled

---

* The *Penny* or *Denny* (denarius?) or *1d.* (in the spoken vernacular, 'one D'—wŭndē') *Council* was officially the Operatives' Committee, a body representing a substantial section of the workmen, clerks and company employees of the region. The 1d. that gave the committee its popular name was the weekly contribution of each subscriber: the aggregate of these weekly pennies met a small but not negligible part of the cost of running the voluntary hospital. In its day the committee did much for the hospital and its patients beyond merely adding to the financial resources. It is no belittlement of the ideals behind the foundation of such councils, or of their positive achievements, to note, if note be needed, that as time passed their membership sometimes tended to include an aggressive, malcontent minority, men who perhaps wanted authority for its own sake and who resented it that the hospital and its staff did not more exclusively serve the rank and file. How wonderfully well served in fact the whole community was, did they but know. Even then. But not more then than now.

at the reasonable proposal that the investigation, which was of no urgency, be put off for a week, until the anaesthetist's return. He was influential as well as opinionated. He had made clear his displeasure at the prospect of what perhaps seemed to him the loss of face before his fellows if he agreed to the postponement of his operation. Still, as he said to the surgeon, if he was not to be admitted on the day originally arranged he would after all be able to attend the next meeting of his committee: and, of course, he would then have to explain to the Brothers why he had been able to be present instead of having his operation, that a doctor had gone on holiday rather than attend to an urgent operation, that only one of the anaesthetists was competent . . . The surgeon gave in, for his absent anaesthetist's appointment on the staff was about due to be renewed, and it was not unknown for the Operatives' Committee to influence such decisions.

So, the surgeon put the committeeman on his list, although it meant he would have to operate under spinal anaesthesia, a procedure that he mistrusted. The spinal anaesthetic was to be given by the first assistant on the surgeon's firm, an experienced advocate of this then comparatively novel method. But when the time for the cystoscopy came the first assistant was himself completing an unexpectedly protracted operation in another hospital. The chief, determined not to put the cystoscopy off, turned to the assistant assistant, whom he knew to have given some 'spinals' under the first assistant's guidance, and told him to do the job.

The patient, a small man of slight build, had marked kyphoscoliosis. Each time the lumbar puncture needle was inserted it hit bone, try as the assistant assistant would to find the right line. The surgeon's presurgical tension began to build up. Soon there appeared the familiar display of studied patience and self-restraint that he had long adopted as protection against reacting too cuttingly when face to face with competence not yet up to his own standards.

After some minutes of watching, in silence except for occasional grunts of patient disapproval and some loud and not quite natural sighs, the surgeon turned his back on the almost desperate manipulations of his sweating colleague and explained to the audience of students what the proposed cystoscopy was for. 'But before the cystoscope is passed the patient must be anaesthetized—that is what Dr——— is trying to do. You will observe the difficulties, gentlemen: Dr——— seems to find his lumbar puncture needle more difficult to pass than I shall find the cystoscope to be, so you will appreciate that a lumbar puncture is not always simple to do, though one may learn by experience, if one has talent. Dr——— is certainly getting the experience . . .'

Worse to the assistant assistant than the humiliation that he felt was his awareness that his chief referred to no would-be surgeon as 'Doctor'—the reversion from 'Mister' to 'Doctor' in these public strictures could only signify that his surgical career was already over. But he kept his mind on what he was trying to do. He withdrew the needle for a fresh start. Putting it in again, again he hit bone. Yet again he withdrew the needle and tried in a slightly different direction. This time he felt only a momentary resistance to the needle before it passed the obstruction. With relief he had found and pierced the spinal theca, he thought, rather deeper and more to the side than expected, the guide-lines distorted by the scoliosis. When he pulled the stylet from the needle no fluid appeared: but, confident now, he attached a syringe and gently pulled on its plunger—a few millilitres of opalescent fluid appeared in the barrel.

'What's that?', asked the surgeon, 'Urine? I am the one who is supposed to be doing the cystoscopy, Dr———. Is it urine? Give it me here—let me smell it!' He sniffed with ostentatious caution at what was in the syringe, then continued, sarcastically perhaps, 'I beg your pardon, Doctor, of course I should have known you wouldn't do all my work for me—it's only duodenal juice'. He paused a moment, the concentration in his look stifling the half-sounded titter from the audience, then asked, almost reverently, 'What do you intend, Doctor? Giving Avertin?* You should have told me sooner—I would rather the patient have a little chloroform and ether. Shall we ask one of these gentlemen'—he nodded toward the students—'to give it for you? You have taxed yourself enough already, Dr————.' But it was the assistant assistant who, though disconsolate, competently gave the C & E.

The patient, nicely premedicated, had been oblivious of all that was untoward. He suffered no ill effects, and the cysto-scopy disclosed no trace of recurrence of the vesical papilloma that had been treated by diathermy some months before.

*   *   *

After the operation the surgeon washed his hands in silence, took one of his theatre sister's cigarettes (traditionally provided from her small earnings) and walked out of the theatre for his regular cup of Lapsang Soochong (traditionally provided by his ward sister from her small earnings, and she doubted if he really appreciated its flavour). The swing doors banged behind him, leaving the assistant assistant alone in the bustle of the theatre as the patient was moved back to bed in the ward and the cleaning-up ritual got under way. But the doors opened again and the surgeon stuck his head into the room, 'Come and have a cup of tea', he said to the younger man, 'You've probably earned it, Mr————. Here, give him one of your cigarettes, Sister.'

If Mr———— reads this, now himself a Chief in the same hospital, I wonder if he will remember the occasion. I think he will.

---

* Avertin, at that time Bayer Products' name for bromethol. Basal anaesthetic. Given rectally.

Comment

Any one who doubts, as I did, that the duodenum can be tapped from behind with a standard lumbar puncture needle should be persuaded of the feasibility of this operation by a simple demonstration on any sparely built, scoliotic cadaver.

Postscript. The fluid that the assistant assistant aspirated through the lumbar puncture needle was shown by the laboratory to be indeed duodenal contents.

50 Needle Biopsy

A man of 55 was found during a periodical health check to have a moderate enlargement of the liver. He had no symptoms. There was no other clinical abnormality and the results of liver function tests were normal. It was decided to do a liver biopsy.

The operation, under local anaesthesia, was carried out with the Menghini needle. The physician who did it and his assistants were used to working together and followed the procedure that they were familiar with, from many scores of similar investigations. Just after the needle had been run into the liver the patient coughed once, sharply. Immediately, he felt acute pain in the right side and shoulder, causing him to go tense and double up before those helping at the operation could restrain him. Within moments he complained of

severe abdominal pain, and collapsed. It was soon clear that
he was bleeding internally.

Immediate laparotomy showed at least a litre of blood in
the peritoneal cavity. There was a deep tear, about six centimetres long, in the lateral aspect of the liver, corresponding
to the plane of the needle puncture. Attempts to suture the
tear failed as the threads cut through the unusually friable
substance of the liver, causing the blood loss to increase.
Eventually, the surgeon managed to control the bleeding by
plugging the rent with large gauze packs, which were removed at a later operation. After a succession of postoperative
complications (biliary peritonitis, secondary haemorrhage,
infective peritonitis, and lung abscess following collapse of
the right lower lobe) the patient recovered and returned to
his administrative job in the hospital service. He has kept well.

In the excitement of the emergency no one remembered to
save the object of it all, the biopsy specimen—by the time it
was thought of one of the theatre juniors had cleaned the
needle. The cause of the enlargement of the liver was never
discovered.

Mutatis mutandis . . . The only other serious misadventure I
have come across in connexion with needle biopsy of the
liver was an acutely fatal haemorrhage in a case of amyloidosis.
The patient was a man of 56 whose liver was found to be
considerably enlarged when he had a routine check of his
fitness to continue his work as an international motor coach
driver. His general condition was remarkably good and he
had no symptoms other than a 'smoker's cough'. Yet X-
raying his chest showed cavitation of the apex of each lung.
There were tubercle bacilli in his sputum. His urine contained
abundant albumin. The clinical diagnosis was amyloidosis
complicating chronic pulmonary phthisis. No amyloid was
found in biopsy specimens of rectal mucosa and gum. It was
decided to do a liver biopsy: this confirmed the diagnosis, at

the cost of his life—like the hospital administrator, he could not suppress a cough that caused the needle to gash the liver. He bled to death before anything could be done to stop it.

Truism. Liver biopsy is not an investigation to be undertaken lightly. What is?

50 + 1 'Curiosa et Exotica'

The Story of an Academic Carrot

is told in the Introduction to the second of the three books in this series, *Exotica*, though whether there will be a chance to read it depends on *your* interest (and the only way we have of judging that will be the sales of *Curiosa* . . .).

Index

An asterisk [*] or dagger [†] indicates that the subject is referred to in a footnote on the corresponding page.

'*Chap.*' indicates that the chapter indicated is primarily or largely concerned with the subject.

'*Fig.*' indicates that the subject is illustrated in the corresponding picture, or, when the number of the figure is followed by the word '*caption*', that the subject is mentioned in the caption.